National Plan for Health Workforce Well-Being

National Academy of Medicine

Action Collaborative on
Clinician Well-Being and Resilience

NATIONAL ACADEMIES PRESS
Washington, DC

NATIONAL ACADEMIES PRESS 500 Fifth Street, NW Washington, DC 20001

This publication has undergone peer review according to procedures established by the National Academy of Medicine (NAM). Publication by the NAM signifies that it is the product of a carefully considered process and is a contribution worthy of public attention but does not constitute endorsement of conclusions and recommendations by the NAM. The views presented in this publication are those of individual contributors and do not represent formal consensus positions of the authors' organizations; the NAM; or the National Academies of Sciences, Engineering, and Medicine.

International Standard Book Number-13: 978-0-309-69467-4
International Standard Book Number-10: 0-309-69467-1
Digital Object Identifier: https://doi.org/10.17226/26744
Library of Congress Catalog Number: 2022918777

Copyright 2024 by the National Academy of Sciences. National Academies of Sciences, Engineering, and Medicine and National Academies Press and the graphical logos for each are all trademarks of the National Academy of Sciences. All rights reserved.

Printed in the United States of America.

Suggested citation: National Academy of Medicine. 2024. National Plan for Health Workforce Well-Being. V. J. Dzau, D. Kirch, V. Murthy, and T. Nasca, editors. NAM Special Publication. Washington, DC: The National Academies Press. https://doi.org/10.17226/26744.

"Knowing is not enough; we must apply.
Willing is not enough; we must do."
-GOETHE

LEADERSHIP
INNOVATION
IMPACT

for a healthier future

ABOUT THE NATIONAL ACADEMY OF MEDICINE

The National Academy of Medicine is one of three Academies constituting the National Academies of Sciences, Engineering, and Medicine (the National Academies). The National Academies provide independent, objective analysis and advice to the nation and conduct other activities to solve complex problems and inform public policy decisions. The National Academies also encourage education and research, recognize outstanding contributions to knowledge, and increase public understanding in matters of science, engineering, and medicine.

The National Academy of Sciences was established in 1863 by an Act of Congress, signed by President Lincoln, as a private, nongovernmental institution to advise the nation on issues related to science and technology. Members are elected by their peers for outstanding contributions to research. Dr. Marcia McNutt is president.

The National Academy of Engineering was established in 1964 under the charter of the National Academy of Sciences to bring the practices of engineering to advising the nation. Members are elected by their peers for extraordinary contributions to engineering. Dr. John L. Anderson is president.

The National Academy of Medicine (formerly the Institute of Medicine) was established in 1970 under the charter of the National Academy of Sciences to advise the nation on issues of health, health care, and biomedical science and technology. Members are elected by their peers for distinguished contributions to medicine and health. Dr. Victor J. Dzau is president.

Learn more about the National Academy of Medicine at NAM.edu.

ACTION COLLABORATIVE ON CLINICIAN WELL-BEING AND RESILIENCE

Steering Committee (2022)

VICTOR J. DZAU (Collaborative Co-Chair), National Academy of Medicine
DARRELL G. KIRCH (Collaborative Co-Chair), Association of American Medical Colleges and Stanford University
VIVEK H. MURTHY (Collaborative Co-Chair), U.S. Department of Health and Human Services
THOMAS J. NASCA (Collaborative Co-Chair), Accreditation Council for Graduate Medical Education
ROBYN BEGLEY, American Hospital Association
DON BERWICK, Institute for Healthcare Improvement
KATIE BOSTON-LEARY, American Nurses Association
ROBERT CAIN, American Association of Colleges of Osteopathic Medicine
PAMELA CIPRIANO, University of Virginia School of Nursing and American Nurses Association
CAROLYN CLANCY, Veterans Health Administration
ERNEST J. GRANT, American Nurses Association
BRETT KESSLER, American Dental Association
LUCINDA L. MAINE, American Association of Colleges of Pharmacy
RICK POLLACK, American Hospital Association
BARRY RUBIN, Peter Munk Cardiac Centre, Toronto General Hospital
LEWIS G. SANDY, UnitedHealth Group
TAIT SHANAFELT, Stanford Medicine
RACHEL VILLANUEVA, National Medical Association
MICHELLE A. WILLIAMS, Harvard T.H. Chan School of Public Health

Action Collaborative Members

NANCY H. AGEE, Carilion Clinic
MEGAN AMAYA, The Ohio State University College of Nursing
ELISA ARESPACOCHAGA, American Hospital Association
DAVID BAKER, The Joint Commission
ALAN BALCH, Patient Advocate Foundation
CONNIE BARDEN, American Association of Critical-Care Nurses
KARI SUE BERNARD, American Academy of PAs Task Force on PA Burnout

CAROL A. BERNSTEIN, Albert Einstein College of Medicine/Montefiore Medical Center
JENNIFER BICKEL, Moffitt Cancer Center
ANDREA BORONDY KITTS, Rescue Lung Society
LEE DAUGHERTY BIDDISON, Johns Hopkins Medicine
STEVE BIRD, UMass Chan Medical School
TIMOTHY BRIGHAM, Accreditation Council for Graduate Medical Education
KIRK J. BROWER, University of Michigan
HELEN BURSTIN, Council of Medical Specialty Societies
NEIL BUSIS, Department of Neurology, NYU Langone Health
PASCALE CARAYON, University of Wisconsin–Madison
MARCELA DEL CARMEN, Massachusetts General Hospital
CHRISTINE CASSEL, University of California, San Francisco
CHIA-CHIA CHANG, CDC National Institute for Occupational Safety and Health
ROBERT A. CHERRY, UCLA Health System
LINDA HAWES CLEVER, RENEW
KEVIN COCKROFT, Penn State Health
MICHAEL F. COLLINS, UMass Chan Medical School
ELISHA DANMEIER, RENEW
SARAH DELGADO, American Association of Critical-Care Nurses
VANESSA DOWNING, ChristianaCare
LOTTE DYRBYE, University of Colorado School of Medicine
HEATHER FARLEY, ChristianaCare
JORDYN FEINGOLD, Icahn School of Medicine at Mount Sinai
SUSAN FORNERIS, National League for Nursing
JESSICA FRIED, University of Michigan
JEANE GARCIA-DAVIS, Office of the Surgeon General
SANDY GOEL, University of Michigan
JEFFERY P. GOLD, University of Nebraska Medical Center
THOMAS GRANATIR, American Board of Medical Specialties
HEATHER GUNNELL, Dartmouth-Hitchcock Medical Center
ROBERT E. HARBAUGH, Penn State Health
RICHARD HAWKINS, American Board of Medical Specialties
ART HENGERER, Federation of State Medical Boards
AMY HILDRETH, Atrium Health Wake Forest Baptist Health
SUSAN HINGLE, SIU School of Medicine and American College of Physicians
EVE HOOVER, American Academy of PAs
KEITH HORVATH, Association of American Medical Colleges
DAVID B. HOYT, American College of Surgeons

LISA ISHII, Johns Hopkins Health System
JAY (JULIUS A.) KAPLAN, LCMC Health and American College of
    Emergency Physicians
JOE KERSCHNER, Medical College of Wisconsin
ANDREA BORONDY KITTS, Rescue Lung Society
BAYLI LARSON, American Society of Health-System Pharmacists
ANNA LEGREID DOPP, American Society of Health-System
    Pharmacists
COLLEEN LENERS, American Association of Colleges of Nursing
SAUL LEVIN, American Psychiatric Association
LORNA LYNN, American Board of Internal Medicine
MICHAEL MAGUIRE, ChristianaCare and Alfred I. duPont Hospital
    for Children
ADITI MALLICK, The George Washington University Hospital
BEVERLY MALONE, National League for Nursing
BARRY MARX, Centers for Medicare and Medicaid Services
BERNADETTE MELNYK, The Ohio State University
DAVID MEYERS, Agency for Healthcare Research and Quality
EDITH MITCHELL, National Medical Association
AMY NGUYEN HOWELL, Optum
LOIS MARGARET NORA, Northeast Ohio Medical University
LAVONNE ORTEGA, Centers for Disease Control and Prevention
NISHA PATEL, UAB Medicine
STACEY PAUL, The Joint Commission
HAL PAZ, Stony Brook University
LAUREN PECCORALO, Icahn School of Medicine at Mount Sinai
JESSICA PERLO, Institute for Healthcare Improvement
THOMAS M. PRISELAC, Cedars-Sinai Health System
DAVID S. RAIFORD, Vanderbilt University Medical Center
NIKHIL RAJAPURAM, Icahn School of Medicine at Mount Sinai
JOHN R. RAYMOND, SR., The Medical College of Wisconsin
RICHARD RIGGS, Cedars-Sinai Health System
JON RIPP, Icahn School of Medicine at Mount Sinai and CHARM
DAVID A. ROGERS, UAB Medicine
JOE ROTELLA, American Academy of Hospice and Palliative
    Medicine
LUKE SATO, CRICO
MARGARET (GRETCHEN) SCHWARZE, University of Wisconsin–
    Madison
JULIE SEES, American Osteopathic Association
SRIJAN SEN, University of Michigan
TINA SHAH, TNT Health Enterprises, LLC
ROBERT SIMARI, University of Kansas Medical Center

STEVE SINGER, Accreditation Council for Continuing Medical Education
CHRISTINE SINSKY, American Medical Association
CYNTHIA (DAISY) SMITH, American College of Physicians
SONYA G. SMITH, American Dental Education Association
KEVIN SOWERS, Johns Hopkins Health System and Johns Hopkins Medicine
MARLO STEIRER, American Board of Medical Specialties
JAVEED SUKHERA, Institute of Living and Hartford Hospital
V. FAN TAIT, American Academy of Pediatrics
CHRISTINE TODD, SIU School of Medicine
TERRY TSUE, University of Kansas Health System
MARK UPTON, Veterans Health Administration
AMY VINSON, American Society of Anesthesiologists and Harvard Medical School
DAVID WEISSMAN, CDC National Institute for Occupational Safety and Health
ERIC WEISSMAN, Association of American Medical Colleges
AMY WINDOVER, Center for Excellence in Healthcare Communication, Cleveland Clinic

Development of this publication was facilitated by the contributions of the following people:

NAM Staff

KIMBER BOGARD, Deputy Executive Officer, Programs
T. ANH TRAN, Program Officer and Director
FARIDA AHMED, Associate Program Officer (from June 2022)
CATHERINE COLGAN, Research Assistant
SAMANTHA PHILLIPS, Communications Officer
JENNA L. OGILVIE, Deputy Director, Communications

Consultant
CHARLEE ALEXANDER, Independent Consultant

REVIEWERS

The products that compose this volume were reviewed in draft form by individuals chosen for their diverse perspectives and technical expertise, in accordance with review procedures established by the National Academy of Medicine (NAM).

We wish to thank the following individuals for their contributions:

> RUMAY ALEXANDER, University of North Carolina at Chapel Hill School of Nursing and American Nurses Association's National Commission Addressing Racism in Nursing
> RICHARD BOTTNER, Colorado Hospital Association
> JESSICA PERLO, Institute for Healthcare Improvement
> KEVIN SOWERS, Johns Hopkins Health System and Johns Hopkins Medicine
> MARK UPTON, Veterans Health Administration

The reviewers listed above provided many constructive comments and suggestions, but they were not asked to endorse the content of the publication and did not see the final draft before it was published. Review of this publication was overseen by KIMBER BOGARD, Deputy Executive Officer, Programs; T. ANH TRAN, Program Officer and Director; FARIDA AHMED, Associate Program Officer; and CATHERINE COLGAN, Research Assistant. Responsibility for the final content of this publication rests entirely with the editors and the NAM.

CONTENTS

Definitions, xiii

Figure and Tables, xvii

Acronyms and Abbreviations, xix

Introduction, 1

1 Priority Area: Create and Sustain Positive Work and Learning Environments and Culture, 9

2 Priority Area: Invest in Measurement, Assessment, Strategies, and Research, 19

3 Priority Area: Support Mental Health and Reduce Stigma, 25

4 Priority Area: Address Compliance, Regulatory, and Policy Barriers for Daily Work, 35

5 Priority Area: Engage Effective Technology Tools, 43

6 Priority Area: Institutionalize Well-Being as a Long-Term Value, 51

7 Priority Area: Recruit and Retain a Diverse and Inclusive Health Workforce, 59

Summary and Conclusion, 69

APPENDIXES

A Background on the Clinician Well-Being Collaborative and National Plan Process, 73
B Background from the National Academies Consensus Study Report and Other Reference Materials for the National Plan's Priority Areas, 75
C References, 83

DEFINITIONS

Burnout is a workplace "syndrome characterized by high emotional exhaustion, high depersonalization (e.g., cynicism), and a low sense of personal accomplishment" (NASEM, 2019).

Culture is the "combination of a body of knowledge, a body of belief, and a body of behavior…. This includes personal identification, language, thoughts, communications, actions, customs, beliefs, values, and institutions" (NIH, 2021).

Health equity is the "state in which everyone has the opportunity to attain full health potential and no one is disadvantaged from achieving this potential because of social position or other socially defined circumstance" (NASEM, 2017).

Health systems encompass organizations and people who work to "improve, maintain, or restore the health of individuals and their communities." Health system settings include hospitals, medical practices, urgent care centers, and other places where health workers deliver care and engage in the "prevention and control of communicable disease and health promotion" (WHO, 2007).

Health workforce comprises a range of occupations, including health workers "such as registered nurses, physicians," and allied health professionals, "as well as individuals in health care support roles, such as community health workers," public health workers, "direct support professionals, and caregivers" (HRSA, 2021). "Health workers" is used to encompass the full range of health professionals, and more specific language is used when necessary.

Mental health is a "state of well-being that enables people to cope with the stresses of life, realize their abilities, learn well and work well, and contribute to their community" (WHO, 2022).

Moral distress occurs when an individual faces a dilemma of knowing their ethical responsibility (e.g., the appropriate care for their patients) but is unable to act upon it due to circumstances beyond their control (Morley et al., 2017). Moral injury is related and occurs when individuals are repeatedly engaging with, failing to prevent, or witnessing such dilemmas (Litz et al., 2009).

Positive work and learning environments are safe and healthy, support the well-being of health workers and learners, and foster ethical and meaningful training and practice (NASEM, 2019).

Professional well-being is a "function of being satisfied with one's job, finding meaning in work, feeling engaged at work, having a high-quality working life, and finding professional fulfillment in work" (Danna and Griffin, 1999; Doble and Santha, 2008).

Psychological safety is a climate of trust and respect in which people are comfortable expressing and being themselves, and share the belief that teammates will not embarrass, reject, or punish a colleague for speaking up (AMA, 2020; Center for Creative Leadership, 2022; Edmonson, 2018).

Resilience is the ability of an individual, organization, "community, or system to withstand, adapt, recover, rebound, or grow from adversity, stress, or trauma" (NASEM, 2019).

Social determinants of health are "the conditions in which people are born, grow, work, live, and age, and the wider set of forces and systems shaping the conditions of daily life." These non-medical factors create socially-defined circumstances that can influence health outcomes (WHO, 2008).

Stigma is a "negative social attitude attached to a characteristic of an individual that may be regarded as a mental, physical, or social deficiency. A stigma implies social disapproval and can lead unfairly to discrimination against and exclusion of the individual" (APA, 2022).

Workplace stress is the "harmful physical and emotional responses that occur when the requirements of the job do not match the capabilities, resources, or needs of the worker. Workplace stress can lead to poor health or even injury" (NIOSH, 2016).

FIGURE AND TABLES

Figure

1   Clinician Well-Being Collaborative Systems Map, 7

Tables

1   Create and Sustain Positive Work and Learning Environments and Culture, 12
2   Invest in Measurement, Assessment, Strategies, and Research, 21
3   Support Mental Health and Reduce Stigma, 28
4   Address Compliance, Regulatory, and Policy Barriers for Daily Work, 37
5   Engage Effective Technology Tools, 45
6   Institutionalize Well-Being as a Long-Term Value, 53
7   Recruit and Retain a Diverse and Inclusive Health Workforce, 62

ACRONYMS AND ABBREVIATIONS

AMA	American Medical Association
CDC	Centers for Disease Control and Prevention
CMS	Centers for Medicare & Medicaid Services
COVID-19	coronavirus disease 2019
CPT	Current Procedural Terminology
EHR	electronic health record
FSMB	Federation of State Medical Boards
HHS	U.S. Department of Health and Human Services
HRSA	Health Resources and Services Administration
IT	information technology
LGBTQIA+	lesbian, gay, bisexual, transgender, queer/questioning, intersex, and ally/asexual
NAM	National Academy of Medicine
NIH	National Institutes of Health
NIOSH	National Institute for Occupational Safety and Health
PPE	personal protective equipment
PTSD	posttraumatic stress disorder
SDOH	social determinants of health
WHO	World Health Organization

Introduction

Health systems do not exist in isolation. Political, market, professional, and cultural forces heavily influence health care delivery, workplace stress, and health worker professional well-being. For decades, health workers have been reporting a loss of meaning in work due to overwhelming job demands and limited supportive resources in the environments in which they operate (Maslach, 2018). In the United States, up to 54 percent of nurses and physicians, 60 percent of medical students and residents, and 61 to 75 percent of pharmacists have symptoms of burnout—high emotional exhaustion, depersonalization (e.g., cynicism), or a low sense of personal accomplishment from work (Jones et al., 2017; NASEM, 2019; Patel et al., 2021). Burnout is a longstanding issue and a fundamental barrier to professional well-being. It was further exacerbated by the coronavirus disease 2019 (COVID-19) pandemic. Health workers who find joy, fulfillment, and meaning in their work can engage on a deeper level with their patients, who are at the heart of health care (Lai et al., 2022; NASEM, 2019). Thus, a thriving workforce is essential for delivering safe, high-quality, patient-centered care.

While the challenge of sustaining the health workforce predated the pandemic, health care teams, including allied health professionals and health care support workers, as well as public health workers, experienced fear while responding to COVID-19—for their personal safety, contracting COVID-19 and spreading it to others, and feeling inadequately prepared to save lives as patients died from a previously unknown disease. They experienced extreme mental and physical fatigue, isolation, and moral and traumatic distress and injury (NAM, 2022a). In April 2020, the death of Dr. Lorna Breen, an emergency physician in New York City, captured national attention and galvanized political action; many members of the public could clearly see the toll on health workers during the COVID-19 pandemic (Knoll et al., 2020).

The pandemic forced the nation to broaden its understanding of the external environment's effects on health delivery and health worker well-being. Early in the pandemic, the world witnessed how health worker physical and emotional well-being was affected by a lack of personal protective equipment (PPE), long hours, and a lack of real-time data to inform clinical decision making. Changing policies at the federal and state levels were critical to adjusting procedures at the organizational level to save lives, though inadequate communication sometimes led to confusion (AAOS, n.d.; Archambault, 2022). Moreover, the public's behaviors seemed to be driven by political ideologies that led to tensions over masks and physical distancing (Hardy et al., 2021). According to multiple surveys of health workers, tensions related to COVID-19 escalated to bullying, harassment, threats, and violence against health workers at work and online (Larkin, 2021). Trust and respect between the public and health workers eroded, ultimately threatening the health workforce's contract with society—dedication to serving the interests of patients while maintaining the public's trust and respect for health workers.

The inequalities that were exacerbated by the pandemic extended to health care environments. Black and Latino/a health workers reported the highest stress levels during the pandemic when compared to White workers (Berg, 2021). This was fueled in part by a greater fear of exposure to COVID-19, since racial and ethnic minority groups disproportionately comprised "essential workers" and other frontline care positions, and were therefore at greater risk of getting sick and dying from COVID-19. Asian and Pacific Islander health workers also reported high stress levels fueled by the pandemic and anti-Asian hate expressed via slurs and physical assaults (Yi, 2020). At a National Academy of Medicine (NAM) convening on unifying the health workforce in March 2022, experts further highlighted the unequal distribution of the burdens placed on certain groups of health workers (see Appendix B for more details on this convening).

While all health worker groups experienced challenges during the pandemic, the emotional well-being of health workers of color were disproportionately affected by COVID-19-related workplace bias, discrimination, and harassment from patients, superiors, and co-workers (NAM, 2022a). One of the first studies to quantify the interplay of individual factors (such as race) with work environmental factors found that nurses of color were hit hard—they reported "higher emotional distress, more negative racial climates, more racial microaggressions, and higher levels of COVID worry" compared to White nurses (Thomas-Hawkins et al., 2022).

Women of color also occupy the majority of jobs, such as nursing assistants and home health aides, in the United States that faced direct occupational and safety risks from lack of protective measures and equipment (CAP, 2020; UNHR, 2020). As schools, daycares, and elder-care facilities closed, female health workers were more often affected by additional caregiving responsibilities compared to their male counterparts (CAP, 2020; NAM, 2022b). Female health workers also reported more work-home conflicts during the pandemic in addition to existing gender-based differences suggested in multiple studies (Templeton et al., 2019; NAM, 2022b).

The resulting severe health workforce shortage, beyond pre-pandemic projections and most critically among nurses, health aides, and assistants, places an enormous burden on remaining health workers and jeopardizes the health of the nation (AHA, 2021; Frogner and Dill, 2022). Before the pandemic, societal costs attributable to health worker burnout in the United States were estimated at $4.6 billion (NASEM, 2019). The costs will only grow, as recent surveys showed high-stress work environments are driving more physicians (20 percent) and nurses (40 percent) to leave practice after two years of the pandemic (Abbasi, 2022). In addition, more than 25 percent of employees in state and local public health departments indicated they are considering leaving their organizations, which exacerbates an already dire situation, as the public health workforce has lost 20 percent of workers since 2008 (de Beaumont, 2021; Stone et al., 2021).

TAKING COLLECTIVE ACTION FOR THE FUTURE OF THE NATION'S HEALTH SYSTEM

> The National Plan's vision is that patients are cared for by a health workforce that is thriving in an environment that fosters their well-being as they improve population health, enhance the care experience, reduce costs, and advance health equity, therefore achieving the quintuple aim.

Collective action is urgently needed to prevent a dissolution of the health professions and to ensure a strong and interconnected health system for the nation. Health workers have been operating in a survival state for a long time, but change is possible. Therefore, an important step is a well-coordinated plan that provides the government, health systems leadership and governance, payers, industry, education, health workers, and leaders in other sectors with the tools and approaches required to drive policy and structural changes.[1] As members of the NAM's Action Collaborative on Clinician Well-Being and Resilience[2] have learned from numerous leading studies and reports, the solution is to take a systems approach that recognizes that no single variable in the health system is to blame for the problem of burnout. Addressing the issue from multiple angles is necessary to redesign environments, so that patients are met with a thriving health workforce that approaches them with all of the skills, expertise, care, and attention they have at their disposal (NASEM, 2019). Leaders have tremendous responsibility and opportunity to address systems issues at the root of workplace stress and burnout. Reducing burnout and moral distress are not enough to achieve professional well-being, though addressing the factors contributing to burnout is fundamental to fostering professional well-being and a thriving health workforce.

This National Plan for Health Workforce Well-Being (National Plan) is intended to inspire collective action that focuses on chang-

---
[1] The chapters that follow list key actors responsible for taking action toward key goals. These lists are not exhaustive. Many of the actors named in this National Plan will need to plan and coordinate their actions with each other as part of a systems approach to health workforce well-being.
[2] For background on the NAM Clinician Well-Being Collaborative, see Appendix A.

es needed across the health system and at the organizational level to improve the well-being of the health workforce. As a nation, we must redesign how health is delivered so that human connection is strengthened, health equity is achieved, and trust is restored. Health delivery can be less transactional and instead center relationships. Our nation should strengthen the public health system and re-invest in the public health infrastructure so that leaders and decision-makers are using the best data and evidence to guide policies locally and across the United States. We need to make investments in the health system, not solely for a financial return on investment, but to improve health delivery and for the long-term well-being of our society. Together, we can create a health system in which care is delivered joyfully and with meaning, by a committed team of all who work to advance health, in partnership with engaged patients and communities.

The National Plan's vision is that patients are cared for by a health workforce that is thriving in an environment that fosters their well-being as they improve population health, enhance the care experience, reduce costs, and advance health equity, therefore achieving the "quintuple aim."[3]

PRIORITIES OF THE NATIONAL PLAN

The National Plan addresses seven priority areas, each focusing on the immediate and long-term needs of the health workforce with the intention that the goals and actions will enable a sustained state of well-being. Each chapter is devoted to discussing a priority area in detail. These priorities strongly echo recommendations from the Taking Action Against Clinician Burnout: A Systems Approach to Professional Well-Being report,[4] as this plan builds on that work and incorporates early lessons and considerations from the COVID-19 pandemic. The seven priorities include:

---

[3] The "quintuple aim" framework to optimize health system performance and care delivery includes advancing health equity and professional well-being as an imperative to (1) improving population health, (2) improving the care experience, and (3) reducing costs (Nundy et al., 2022).

[4] For information on the National Academies' consensus study report and foundational materials to the National Plan's priority areas, see Appendix B. Find the full National Academies' consensus study report at: National Academies of Sciences, Engineering, and Medicine (NASEM). 2019. Taking Action Against Clinician Burnout: A Systems Approach to Professional Well-Being. Washington, DC: The National Academies Press. https://doi.org/10.17226/25521.

- Create and sustain positive work and learning environments and culture. Transform health systems, health education, and training by prioritizing and investing in efforts to optimize environments that prevent and reduce burnout, foster professional well-being, and support quality care (NASEM, 2019).
- Invest in measurement, assessment, strategies, and research. Expand the uptake of existing tools at the health system level and advance national research on decreasing health worker burnout and improving well-being.
- Support mental health and reduce stigma. Provide support to health workers by eliminating barriers and reducing stigma associated with seeking services needed to address mental health challenges.
- Address compliance, regulatory, and policy barriers for daily work. Prevent and reduce the unnecessary burdens that stem from laws, regulations, policies, and standards placed on health workers.
- Engage effective technology tools. Optimize and expand the use of health information technologies that support health workers in providing high-quality patient care and serving population health, and minimize technologies that inhibit clinical decision-making or add to administrative burden.
- Institutionalize well-being as a long-term value. Ensure COVID-19 recovery efforts address the toll on health worker well-being now and in the future, and bolster the public health and health care systems for future emergencies.
- Recruit and retain a diverse and inclusive health workforce. Promote careers in the health professions and increase pathways and systems for a diverse, inclusive, and thriving workforce.

Transforming the U.S. health system is a complex challenge, and imagining the journey toward a thriving health workforce can be daunting. Nevertheless, important steps continue to be made. For example, following the death of Dr. Lorna Breen, her family rallied policymakers and other key stakeholders to successfully lead the passage of the Dr. Lorna Breen Health Care Provider Protection Act in 2022, which begins to support the mental and behavioral health

Introduction | 7

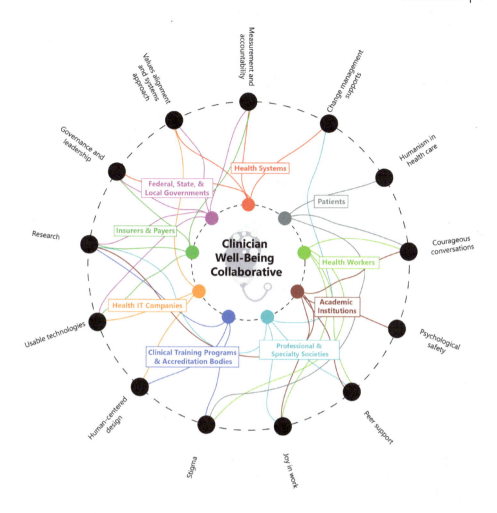

Figure 1 | Clinician Well-Being Collaborative Systems Map
NOTES: This figure depicts the actors (inner ring) who participated in the Clinician Well-Being Collaborative's work (outer ring) from 2017 to 2022, to ultimately make progress toward clinician well-being. These and additional actor groups are called upon in this National Plan to drive systems change through collective action.
SOURCE: Adapted from National Academy of Medicine, 2020.

of health workers (117th Congress, 2021). This is a major indicator of progress toward a health system that better serves both patients and health workers.

Everyone—from health workers to the public to multi-sectoral leaders—has a role in tackling health workforce well-being (see Figure 1).

However, in the wake of COVID-19 and its impacts on the health workforce, the nation is experiencing a cultural shift, where every actor must take ownership of their role and join in building a social movement for health workforce well-being (Kahan and Avritt, 2015). This National Plan is a crucial component that will help coordinate actions across the field and provide a roadmap for developing a system of accountability to monitor efforts and track progress on advancing health worker well-being. Through the collective work among organizations and individuals committed to reversing trends in health worker burnout, particularly over the past six years, many of the foundational pieces are in place to begin a social movement to advance health worker well-being.[5]

The priorities, goals, and actions laid out in the National Plan are urgent and complex. No single actor or sector can move the needle on its own, and change will not happen overnight. But such complexity cannot be an excuse for inaction. Every actor and sector should identify the most pressing priorities or promising opportunities and develop plans for near-, medium-, and long-term actions in accordance with available resources and in collaboration with other actors. This is difficult work, but we must remain collectively committed.

Now is the time to re-establish the social contract between health workers and society. This mutual agreement and understanding calls on health workers to fulfill their roles as healers. In exchange, society grants trust in the health professions, provides the ability for professions to self-govern, and shares in the responsibility for improving public health and maintaining health infrastructure and systems (Khan et al., 2022). The health of the nation depends on it.

---

[5] Adapting the work of Kahan and Avritt (2015), the 10 key elements for creating a social movement for health worker well-being are (1) the burnout and COVID-19 crises, (2) science-based research on burnout and well-being, (3) economics of addressing burnout, (4) spark plug actors to drive social change, (5) coalition building, (6) advocacy, (7) government involvement, (8) mass communication, (9) environmental and policy change, and (10) a national plan. The NAM Clinician Well-Being Collaborative has made progress in many of these elements over the past 6 years.

1

Priority Area: Create and Sustain Positive Work and Learning Environments and Culture

Transform health systems, health education, and training by prioritizing and investing in efforts to optimize environments that prevent and reduce burnout, foster professional well-being, and support quality care (NASEM, 2019).

"Invest in and prioritize a true well-being program and prioritize it to make it a culture. Often organizational policies and expectations are conflicting with true commitment to well-being. There needs to be more than just telling people to take care of themselves."
- Frontline Health Worker[1]

Positive work and learning environments for health workers are intertwined with safe environments for patient care and population health. Not only is it part of an organization's ethical responsibility to invest in health worker well-being, but evidence also suggests that it is central to optimizing patient outcomes and addressing costs associated with staff turnover, lost revenue, financial risk, and threats to a health system's long-term viability (Shanafelt et al., 2017). However, there is no one-size-fits-all solution to improving health worker well-being, and there are challenges for organizations and small practices alike in navigating appropriate investments that are reflective of their local context. For health systems,

---
[1] For background on this quote and those in other chapters, visit the NAM's Clinician Burnout Crisis in the Era of COVID-19: Insights from the Frontlines of Care webpage at: https://nam.edu/initiatives/clinician-resilience-and-well-being/clinician-burnout-crisis-in-the-era-of-covid-19/.

changing the environment and culture will require a systems approach of active and engaged executive leadership that meaningfully involves staff throughout the organization, including service line directors, department chairs, clinical learning environment directors, and frontline workers in decision-making, establishing frameworks for holding each other accountable, and fostering a culture of continuous learning and improvement (NASEM, 2019). Strategies to encourage respect among health workers and to combat workplace bullying, abuse, and threats toward health workers are important to prevent harm from disrespect in work and learning environments, protect health workers, and ensure workers can focus on delivering care (Sokol-Hessner et al., 2018).

Addressing health worker well-being requires financial, time, and human resource investments, and leaders and health workers must make the case to address well-being when faced with numerous and seemingly competing challenges. Estimates on the cost of turnover, depending on role types, range from $88,000 to more than $1 million to replace a registered nurse or physician (Dyrbye et al., 2017). Studies point to the potential of burned out and overworked physicians making unnecessary referrals and ordering more tests, and burnout among health workers may raise health expenditures via medical errors, malpractice claims, absenteeism, and lower productivity (Dyrbye et al., 2017). Therefore, emphasizing and addressing well-being is aligned with organizational goals to improve quality care and reduce costs. It is not an additional priority, but rather a central priority, with additive benefits across the health system.

Though optimizing work conditions and managing the workforce were challenges for many health systems, including small and rural practices, before the pandemic, these pressures have only grown more acute. For example, the end of temporary federal assistance for rural hospitals that face closures due to financial challenges will threaten access to much needed health care services for Medicare and Medicaid recipients (Bhatnagar et al., 2022). It is clear that many health systems, from rural to urban and small to large health care delivery organizations, have coped with profound pressure on staff and resources (KaufmanHall, 2022). Work stressors during the COVID-19 pandemic have driven health workers to leave the profession, exacerbating the burdens on remaining staff and perpetuating a cycle of introducing new workers into unhealthy work and learning environments, particularly in rural communities (Wright, 2021). As health systems mitigate critical staffing shortages (e.g., contracting labor to ensure that patient care and organizational operations remain safe), they must also address other factors impacting the workforce and broader society, such as structural racism, sexism, ableism, and anti-LGBTQIA+ (lesbian, gay, bisexual, transgender, queer/questioning, intersex, and ally/asexual) discrimination and bias. Not surprisingly, discrimination and bias affect education, training, and work environments for health workers, with devastating results for patient experiences, perceptions, and outcomes (Leape et al., 2012; Hu et al., 2019; ANA, 2022).

Health workers want to see an enhanced commitment from their organizations to promote diversity, equity, inclusion, and accessibility in the health system in partnership with their communities (NAM, 2022a, 2022b). Diversifying the workforce has the dual benefits of improving patient care experiences and increasing the available staff to provide care. Leaders and health workers can build upon this practice of embracing all health worker identities by practicing cultural humility, "being aware of how an individual's culture can impact their health behaviors and using this awareness to cultivate sensitive approaches in treating patients" (Prasad et al., 2016). It is important to recognize that individuals—from practicing health workers to learners—hail from a range of different backgrounds, experiences, and professional cultures, yet they ultimately come together as a care team. Purposeful interactions celebrating and respecting professional strengths and appreciating personal differences are key to the well-being of both patients and providers.

The consistent and sustainable delivery of safe and high-quality patient care is only possible when clinical learning environments ensure the well-being of all health workers (ACGME, 2019). Executive and educational leaders must partner to foster an enabling culture—the importance of designing solutions to keep pace with the rapidly changing health delivery environment cannot be overstated (Nasca et al., 2014). Significant opportunities remain to optimize care delivery models to leverage technology and advanced analytics (see Chapter 5), team-based principles, and other emerging approaches.

Priority Area: Create and sustain positive work and learning environments and culture.	
Goal 1.1.	Culture of well-being is integrated into program operations, human resource management, services, and curricula.
Actors	Academic Institutions, Clinical Training Programs, and Accreditation Bodies
	Health Systems
	Health Workers
	Insurers and Payers
Actions	1.1.A. Instill approaches to decrease workplace stress and burnout, and improve health worker and learner well-being in strategic plans, organizational values, and human resources policies and procedures.
	1.1.B. Implement well-being onboarding programs for students as they enter health professions schools to build coping and resiliency skills.
	1.1.C. Provide training opportunities for faculty to help integrate well-being into programming.
	1.1.D. Set reasonable productivity expectations and provide adequate resources to support expectations.

Goal 1.2.	Settings are diverse, equitable, accessible, and inclusive.
Actors	Academic Institutions, Clinical Training Programs, and Accreditation Bodies
	Health Information Technology (IT) Companies
	Health Systems
	Health Workers
Actions	1.2.A. Examine institutional policies, organizational goals, and objectives with an equity lens.
	1.2.B. Revise clinical algorithms that erroneously rely on race.
	1.2.C. Establish policies and processes to support the timely reporting of and response to discriminatory behaviors. This includes a clear reporting process, support for reporters, and outcomes commensurate with the demonstrated behavior and situation.
	1.2.D. Establish mentorship programs to help all health workers thrive in educational, training, and practice environments.
	1.2.E. Review leadership opportunities and pathways to ensure they are diverse, accessible, equitable, and inclusive, and are available at multiple levels of a health system and training program.
	1.2.F. Provide appropriate education and trainings for workers, staff, and leaders to address issues (e.g., discrimination, lateral violence, bullying, harassment) and progress toward cultural humility.

Goal 1.3.	There is increased retention and decreased turnover of health workers.	
Actors		Academic Institutions, Clinical Training Programs, and Accreditation Bodies
		Federal, State, and Local Governments
		Health Systems
		Health Workers
		Insurers and Payers
Actions	1.3.A. Provide mechanisms and systems to allow health workers to operate as teams.	
	1.3.B. Invest in appropriate and flexible staffing plans that allow for safe patient care, including needed backup.	
	1.3.C. Create and implement processes for meaningful recognition for all members of the health workforce.	
	1.3.D. Examine sick leave and personal time off policies and staffing to accommodate health workers who need time off, regardless of their tenure.	
	1.3.E. Develop and incentivize coverage systems that allow health workers to take time off, especially so that frontline workers can hand off responsibility for patient care during their time away.	
	1.3.F. Offer employee benefits that include child care and elder care services.	
	1.3.G. Ensure that health worker meal and rest breaks are expected and routine, not exceptional.	
	1.3.H. Learn about health worker experiences directly by asking them and conducting surveys and listening sessions while they are employed, and conducting exit interviews to understand why they are leaving their positions.	
	1.3.I. Promote work-life integration for health workers through structures such as sufficient staff, flexible schedules, access to and use of health care, and low-cost and healthy food options.	
	1.3.J. Address accountability and reward systems to re-orient promotion/tenure and salary processes so that they reward behaviors contributing to positive learning environments.	

Create and Sustain Positive Work and Learning Environments and Culture | 15

Goal 1.4.	Leadership recognizes negative impacts of health worker burnout and fosters a culture of well-being.
Actors	Academic Institutions, Clinical Training Programs, and Accreditation Bodies
	Health Systems
	Health Workers
	Professional and Specialty Societies
Actions	1.4.A. Use data to develop strategies that will continually improve well-being and decrease health worker burnout and distress.
	1.4.B. Ensure that leaders consider well-being when making decisions, to account for the potential impact on patients, the workforce, and their health systems.
	1.4.C. Provide protected time for and empower managers, health workers, and other staff to address well-being in the workplace.
	1.4.D. Invest in well-being leadership roles, such as Chief Wellness Officers (and Chief Nursing and Chief Pharmacy Officers, as appropriate) that: • report to executive leadership and governance and are integrated in the leadership team, • facilitate uptake and accountability of well-being within the heath workforce, and • are allocated the resources necessary to implement strategies that will improve health worker well-being.

Goal 1.5.	Accountability standards and best practices for well-being are adopted.
Actors	Academic Institutions, Clinical Training Programs, and Accreditation Bodies
	Health Systems
	Professional and Specialty Societies
	Private and Non-Profit Organizations
Actions	1.5.A. Establish and implement accountability measures and incentives for leaders (see Action 3J).
	1.5.B. Fund and evaluate demonstration programs and grants in the workplace and learning environments.
	1.5.C. Decrease the amount of time between research and translating evidence into real-world settings.

NOTE: The list of actors in this table is not exhaustive. Many of the actors named in this table will need to plan and coordinate their actions with each other as part of a systems approach to health workforce well-being.

RELATED RESOURCES[2][1]

Advance Organizational Commitment
- White Paper: Framework for Improving Joy in Work (Perlo et al., 2017)
- Report: CLER Pathways to Excellence: Expectations for an Optimal Clinical Learning Environment to Achieve Safe and High-Quality Patient Care, Version 2.0 (Accreditation Council for Graduate Medical Education)
- Guide: Well-Being Playbook: A Guide for Hospital and Health System Leaders (American Hospital Association)

---

[2] For additional resources, visit the NAM's Resource Compendium for Health Care Worker Well-Being webpage at: https://nam.edu/compendium-of-key-resources-for-improving-clinician-well-being/.

- Guide: Establishing a Chief Wellness Officer Position (Shanafelt and Sinsky, 2020b)
- Guide: The Pharmacist's Fundamental Rights and Responsibilities (American Pharmacists Association and the National Alliance of State Pharmacy Associations)
- Guide: NIOSH Safe Patient Handling and Mobility (National Institute for Occupational Safety and Health)
- Case Example: Workplace Wellness Champions: Lessons Learned and Implications for Future Programming (Amaya et al., 2017)
- Infographic: Survey Shows Substantial Racism in Nursing (National Commission to Address Racism in Nursing)
- Recognition Programs:
    - Joy in Medicine Health System Recognition Program (American Medical Association)
    - Beacon Award (American Association of Critical-Care Nurses)
    - Pathway to Excellence Program and the Magnet Recognition Program (American Nurses Credentialing Center)
    - ASHP Certified Center of Excellence in Medication-Use Safety and Pharmacy Practice (American Society of Health-System Pharmacists)

Strengthen Leadership Behaviors
- Guide: Chief Wellness Officer Roadmap (Shanafelt and Sinsky, 2020a)
- Discussion Paper: A Call to Action: Align Well-Being and Antiracism Strategies (Barrett et al., 2021)

Conduct Workplace Assessment
- Overview of Established Tools: Valid and Reliable Survey Instruments to Measure Burnout, Well-Being, and Other Work-Related Dimensions (National Academy of Medicine)
- Infographic/Assessment Tool: Standards for Establishing and Sustaining a Healthy Work Environment (American Association of Critical-Care Nurses)
- Guide: NIOSH Total Worker Health Program (National Institute for Occupational Safety and Health)

Cultivate a Culture of Connection and Support
- Guide: A Nurse's Guide to Preventing Compassion Fatigue, Moral Distress, and Burnout (American Nurses Foundation)
- Guide: "What Matters to You?" Conversation Guide for Improving Joy in Work (Institute for Healthcare Improvement)
- Case Study: Culture of Well-Being (American Hospital Association)

2

Priority Area: Invest in Measurement, Assessment, Strategies, and Research

Expand the uptake of existing tools at the health system level and advance national research on decreasing health worker burnout and improving well-being.

> "So far, most of the response of my organization has been psychosocial support for health care workers, but I'd like to see us measure burnout organizationally, track it and design improvement efforts around it." - Frontline Health Worker[1]

Burnout negatively affects patient outcomes, health workers, and health system finances; high rates of burnout reported by U.S. health workers are a signal that the overall health system is failing to achieve system-wide improvement (NASEM, 2019). The longitudinal use of validated tools is required to accurately measure the prevalence of burnout and distress in health care settings of all sizes and in all locations, as well as the impact of strategies to decrease workplace burnout. Measuring and understanding the drivers of workplace distress and burnout among individuals, and particularly health care teams, are essential to forming the baseline for organizations to establish their well-being guidelines and to evaluating the effectiveness of strategies to decrease workplace distress and improve health worker well-being. However, employing measures that are unable to capture burnout holistically can be inappropriate and do more harm than good (NASEM, 2019).

---

[1] For background on this quote and those in other chapters, visit the NAM's Clinician Burnout Crisis in the Era of COVID-19: Insights from the Frontlines of Care webpage at: https://nam.edu/initiatives/clinician-resilience-and-well-being/clinician-burnout-crisis-in-the-era-of-covid-19/.

Metrics to assess the prevalence of burnout need to be harmonized with organizational efforts around employee engagement and satisfaction. These metrics also need to be appropriate for the setting, using valid and reliable survey instruments to measure burnout, well-being, and other "clinically relevant dimensions of distress that include meaning in work, severe fatigue, work-life integration, quality of life, and suicidal ideation" (Dyrbye et al., 2016). More validation and efforts to assess burnout among health professional students are needed, though burnout surveys for medical students have emerged. Cross-walks between workplace measures of burnout and distress have also been developed (Brady et al., 2022). For health systems, the choice of which survey to implement matters less than the decision to choose a validated survey tool and the commitment to measure and report the prevalence of health worker burnout and distress over time. Accurate assessment of total workload and the quality of care provides complementary data to surveys of burnout and distress, and should also be regularly included (Sinsky et al., 2020). At the national level, additional research is needed to not only better understand the extent of health worker burnout as a baseline but also to identify links to clinical outcomes, and ultimately build on the success of various interventions for decreasing burnout and improving well-being across the field.

Importantly, data that identify the prevalence of health workforce burnout should not be used for public rankings due to the highly subjective nature of the questions and undue incentives to receive high scores, rather than to collect honest feedback for internal use to drive change (Mayer et al., 2021; NASEM, 2019). As mentioned in Chapter 1, it is in an organization's financial interests and part of their care responsibility to take action to decrease burnout among health workers, but other actor groups can take shared responsibility and provide additional incentives as part of a systems approach.

Priority Area: Invest in measurement, assessment, strategies, and research.

Goal 2.1.	Burnout and well-being of health workers and learners, and the drivers of workplace stress, are routinely measured.
Actors	Academic Institutions, Clinical Training Programs, and Accreditation Bodies
	Health Systems
	Health Workers
	Insurers and Payers
Actions	2.1.A. Measure and assess core leadership behaviors that promote workforce well-being (e.g., the Mayo Clinic Leader Index uses the Include, Inform, Inquire, Develop, Recognize framework; see Related Resources).
	2.1.B. Identify internal and external funding streams for measurement and assessment of learner and health workforce burnout and well-being.
	2.1.C. Measure the prevalence and drivers of health worker and learner burnout and distress, using one of the existing validated survey tools for which established benchmarks are available.
	2.1.D. Recognize and evaluate the links between well-being outcomes and key performance indicators that are most relevant to the organization and learning environments (e.g., quality of care, patient-reported outcomes and experience, staff turnover).
	2.1.E. Disaggregate and de-identify data, share it across the organization and to relevant groups for the purpose of continuous learning, and use it to develop intervention strategies that will drive positive local changes in the workplace and learning environments.

Goal 2.2.	A national commitment is made to invest in research, strategies, and partnerships to improve health worker and learner well-being.
Actors	Academic Institutions, Clinical Training Programs, and Accreditation Bodies
	Federal, State, and Local Governments
	Health Information Technology (IT) Companies
	Health Systems
	Health Workers
	Insurers and Payers
	Private and Non-Profit Organizations
	Professional and Specialty Societies
Actions	2.2.A. Coordinate a research agenda to examine: • organizational, learning environment, and health system factors (e.g., payment models, health IT, regulatory practices, workload and staffing models, local culture) that contribute to burnout, moral injury, occupational distress, intention to leave health care as a profession, and death by suicide among health workers; • the impact of bias, discrimination, sexism, ableism, anti-LGBTQIA+ (lesbian, gay, bisexual, transgender, queer/questioning, intersex, and ally/asexual) efforts and/or racism on the professional and personal well-being of health workers and learners; • the immediate and long-term effects of COVID-19 on the well-being of the health workforce; and • strategies to improve health worker and learner well-being in the local environment.

Actions	2.2.B. Fund a coordinated research agenda that focuses primarily on the issues outlined in Action 2A.
	2.2.C. Create and manage a national registry of evidence-based interventions to coordinate and facilitate research and innovation aimed at eliminating health worker and learner burnout and improving professional worker and learner well-being.
	2.2.D. Establish and support a national epidemiologic tracking program to measure health worker and learner well-being, distress, and burnout with mandated funding.
	2.2.E. Enhance wide-scale uptake of implementation best practices and approaches to improve well-being and decrease burnout across various stakeholder groups.
	2.2.F. Convene conferences and symposia to share strategies for improving well-being and preventing and reducing burnout and distress.

NOTE: The list of actors in this table is not exhaustive. Many of the actors named in this table will need to plan and coordinate their actions with each other as part of a systems approach to health workforce well-being.

RELATED RESOURCES[2]

Conduct Workplace Assessment
- Overview of Established Tools: Valid and Reliable Survey Instruments to Measure Burnout, Well-Being, and Other Work-Related Dimensions (National Academy of Medicine)
- Tool: Healthy Work Environment Assessment Tool (American Association of Critical-Care Nurses)
- Tool: NIOSH Worker Well-Being Questionnaire (WELLBQ) (National Institute for Occupational Safety and Health)
- Tool: Wellness Culture and Environment Support Scale (Melnyk and Amaya, 2018)
- Calculator: Organizational Cost of Physician Burnout (American Medical Association)
- Discussion Paper: A Pragmatic Approach for Organizations to Measure Health Care Professional Well-Being (Dyrbye et al., 2018)

[2] For additional resources, visit the NAM's Resource Compendium for Health Care Worker Well-Being webpage at: https://nam.edu/compendium-of-key-resources-for-improving-clinician-well-being/.

- Discussion Paper: Establishing Crosswalks Between Common Measures of Burnout in US Physicians (Brady et al., 2022)
- Survey Findings: Pulse on the Nation's Nurses Survey Series: COVID-19 Two-Year Impact Assessment Survey (American Nurses Foundation, 2022)

Strengthen Leadership Behaviors

- Guide: Cultivating Leadership: Measure and Assess Leader Behaviors to Improve Professional Well-Being (American Medical Association)
- Perspective: Preventing a Parallel Pandemic—A National Strategy to Protect Clinicians' Well-Being (Dzau et al., 2020)

3

Priority Area: Support Mental Health and Reduce Stigma

Provide support to health workers by eliminating barriers and reducing stigma associated with seeking services to address mental health challenges.

"We need investment in mental health in the long term, funding and access to care, and change in barriers to access like conversations about care and stigma in our culture."
- Frontline Health Worker[1]

Mental health is a "state of mental well-being that enables people to cope with the stresses of life, realize their abilities, learn well and work well, and contribute to their community" (WHO, 2018). Mental health disorders affect 15 to 20 percent of U.S. adults in any given year and are the leading cause of disability in the country (U.S. Burden of Disease Collaborators, 2013). For health care workers specifically, the nature of their clinical training and work is linked to substantial increases in depression, anxiety, suicidal ideation, and other mental health conditions upon entering the profession, with high rates persisting through their careers (Bellini et al., 2002; Mata et al., 2015; Melnyk et al., 2020). There is a continuum of stress in the environment with multiple phases and implications (Nash et al., 2010). Past pandemics and emerging evidence suggest that many health workers will have experiences along the stress continuum, which could include COVID-19-related trauma,

---

[1] For background on this quote and those in other chapters, visit the NAM's Clinician Burnout Crisis in the Era of COVID-19: Insights from the Frontlines of Care webpage at: https://nam.edu/initiatives/clinician-resilience-and-well-being/clinician-burnout-crisis-in-the-era-of-covid-19/.

posttraumatic stress disorder (PTSD), risk for substance use, and depression (McKay and Asmundson, 2020). Ultimately, if health workers are not well, health care delivery and patient safety may suffer (Fahrenkopf et al., 2008).

There is robust evidence that mental health disorders can be prevented, and prevention approaches have the potential to substantially reduce the public health burden of these disorders (Muñoz et al., 2012). It should be noted that prevention strategies and treatments differ for mental health challenges and problems that are potentially linked with substance use and addiction. Prevention efforts should be aimed at populations, such as health workers and other professionals, where the prevalence of disorders are high and important drivers of poor mental health have been identified. To decrease the number of health workers and learners who develop depression, anxiety, and other mental health issues, it is critical that health systems address the structural challenges that are driving some of their employees' poor mental health, such as high workload, administrative burden, and work-family conflict (Fang et al., 2022; Guille et al., 2017). When mental health issues arise, these upstream drivers must be addressed, in addition to the provision of appropriate mental health resources and referrals. This requires appropriate triage by skilled mental health professionals at the individual level who can distinguish between burnout and mental and behavioral health issues and make an accurate referral for treatment. Health workers struggling with addiction and fearful of losing their licenses should have assistance, since there are significant consequences—not only to themselves but also for their patients—if they remain untreated (Butler Center for Research, 2015).

In the United States, stigma associated with seeking support for emotional and mental health and substance use is widespread in the general population (NASEM, 2019). Negative perceptions, attitudes, and discrimination regarding help-seeking are entrenched in the health professions' culture and training, as well as individual perceptions of and the actual expectations and responses of health systems, licensing bodies, and other governing forces (NASEM, 2019). As such, many mental health programs, even when implemented, face resistance from health workers, so planning for psychological intervention programs should include promotion and awareness campaigns at the organizational level (Buselli et al., 2021). At the state level, despite progress in recent years on updated licensing applications to encourage treatment-seeking among health workers, this stigma continues to be pervasive (FSMB, 2018; Halter et al., 2019).[2] In practice, health workers may still internalize shame, avoid speaking up and getting care, or avoid fully sharing their experiences with their employers. Continuing to eliminate both policy barriers to care and cultural stigma are foundational to the professional well-being of health workers and learners.

---

[2] In 2018, the Federation of State Medical Boards released recommendations for licensing applications to ask only about current impairments to practicing—not all conditions—that might undermine a physician's ability to work safely (FSMB, 2018). These licensing updates would be consistent with the Americans with Disabilities Act, which prohibits discrimination against those with mental health conditions. Many state boards of nursing are also modifying their licensing applications (Halter et al., 2019).

Priority Area: Support mental health and reduce stigma.	
Goal 3.1.	The mental health workforce is strengthened with increased numbers of practitioners.
Actors	Academic Institutions, Clinical Training Programs, and Accreditation Bodies
	Federal, State, and Local Governments
	Health Systems
	Insurers and Payers
	Professional and Specialty Societies
Actions	3.1.A. Train, recruit, and retain additional mental health professionals (e.g. mental health nurse practitioners, occupational therapists, psychiatrists, psychologists, physician assistants, and social workers) to provide care for the health workforce.
	3.1.B. Increase resources to support individuals seeking education to become mental health professionals.
	3.1.C. Continue to address the lack of pay parity between health professionals providing mental health services and those who provide other forms of treatment.
	3.1.D. Establish debt forgiveness programs and pathways to increase the interest of learners in mental health professions.
	3.1.E. Integrate training on referral pathways from primary care to specialty mental health care.

Support Mental Health and Reduce Stigma | 29

Goal 3.2.	Adequate mental health services are available, easily accessible, confidential, dignified, paid for, and health workers and learners are encouraged to use them.
Actors	Federal, State, and Local Governments
	Health Systems
	Health Workers
	Insurers and Payers
	Private and Non-Profit Organizations
	Professional and Specialty Societies
Actions	3.2.A. Provide supportive mental health services for health workers involved in safety events and other traumatic events as part of a system's layered protections against medical errors.
	3.2.B. Support the use of faith leaders, coaches, peer supporters, and other trusted resources due to the shortage of licensed mental health professionals.
	3.2.C. Provide quality mental health services, offer telemedicine and virtual care options where appropriate, and expand hours of availability to when health workers are not at work.
	3.2.D. Offer external providers of mental health services to emphasize confidentiality.
	3.2.E. Arrange coverage and/or flexible schedules for health workers to participate in mental health appointments.
	3.2.F. Establish peer-support programs and offer psychological and/or stress first-aid training for all health workers and trainees, in addition to Employee Assistance Programs.
	3.2.G. Guarantee mental health parity with other medical conditions for the coverage of health care costs.
	3.2.H. Increase reimbursement and reform prior authorization for mental health services to ensure health workers and trainees receive the care they need.

Goal 3.3.	Stigma and barriers are reduced for health workers and learners to disclose mental health issues and utilize mental health services.
Actors	Academic Institutions, Clinical Training Programs, and Accreditation Bodies
	Federal, State, and Local Governments
	Health Systems
	Health Workers
	Media and Communications
	Private and Non-Profit Organizations
	Professional and Specialty Societies
Actions	3.3.A. Increase awareness of mental health issues and services through routine communications, such as rounds or regularly scheduled meetings, and other dissemination efforts.
	3.3.B. Develop policies and exemplar practices regarding requirements for privileging and credentialing in health care delivery organizations.
	3.3.C. Convene state licensing and certification boards to accelerate appropriate changes to mental health reporting requirements, reduce stigma, and normalize the process for health workers to seek help for workplace-related stresses.
	3.3.D. Educate the public and health workforce about the benefits of mentally healthy workers.

Support Mental Health and Reduce Stigma | 31

Goal 3.4.	Health workers and learners do not experience unnecessary punitive actions when seeking mental health services.
Actors	Academic Institutions, Clinical Training Programs, and Accreditation Bodies
	Federal, State, and Local Governments
	Health Systems
	Insurers and Payers
Actions	3.4.A. Align questions about personal health information with the Americans with Disabilities Act to inquire only about current impairments that may affect their ability to provide care due to a health condition rather than a past or current diagnosis or treatment for a mental health condition.
	3.4.B. Establish accountability frameworks for ensuring psychologically safe working and learning environments that prevent discrimination, such as inappropriate retaliation or termination, against health workers and learners disclosing mental health challenges.

Goal 3.5.	Access to mental health resources is correlated with improved health worker well-being.
Actors	Academic Institutions, Clinical Training Programs, and Accreditation Bodies
	Federal, State, and Local Governments
	Health Systems
	Professional and Specialty Societies
Actions	3.5.A. Track the use of mental health services and programs (e.g., Employee Assistance Program) to ensure programs are designed to meet the needs of health workers, whether efforts to seek assistance and treatment have increased, and whether organizational barriers (such as stigma, lack of confidentiality, fear of punitive consequences, etc.) have been removed. NOTE: Data should be de-identified.
	3.5.B. Track whether state-level barriers have been removed.

NOTE: The list of actors in this table is not exhaustive. Many of the actors named in this table will need to plan and coordinate their actions with each other as part of a systems approach to health workforce well-being.

RELATED RESOURCES[3][1]

Cultivate a Culture of Connection and Support
- Organizational Guide: 2022 Healthcare Workforce Rescue Package (National Academy of Medicine and All In)
- Organizational Guide: Conversation and Action Guide to Support Staff Well-Being and Joy in Work During and After the COVID-19 Pandemic (Institute for Healthcare Improvement)
- Organizational Graphic: Psychological PPE: Promote Health Care Workforce Mental Health and Well-Being (Institute for Healthcare Improvement)

---
[3] For additional resources, visit the NAM's Resource Compendium for Health Care Worker Well-Being webpage at: https://nam.edu/compendium-of-key-resources-for-improving-clinician-well-being/.

- Organizational Guide: Peer Support Programs for Physicians (Shapiro, 2020)
- Organizational Guide: At the Heart of the Pandemic: Nursing Peer Support (Godfrey and Scott, 2020)
- Organizational Guide: Preventing Physician Suicide: Identify and Support At-Risk Physicians (Brooks, 2016)
- Individual Support Guide: Provider Well-Being for Behavioral Health Professionals (Mental Health Technology Transfer Center Network)
- Individual Support Guide: Health Care Professionals (National Alliance on Mental Illness)
- Resource Compilation: COVID Resources (American Psychiatric Nurses Association)

4

Priority Area: Address Compliance, Regulatory, and Policy Barriers for Daily Work

Prevent and reduce the unnecessary burdens that stem from laws, regulations, policies, and standards placed on health workers.

"Reduce the regulatory burden which makes health workers feel like data entry people." - Frontline Health Worker[1]

Health workers are faced with time-consuming tasks that detract from time spent with patients or promoting health, and they are often not empowered to take back their time (Sinsky et al., 2020). Though standards are essential to providing safe, high-quality care, the constellation of organizational, state, and federal policies have created administrative requirements that multiply over the course of a health worker's day. Depending on the clarity of guidance from government agencies, overly conservative interpretation of regulations at the organizational level can result in a less safe environment for patient care, as health workers lose time and cognitive bandwidth for clinical care while addressing multiplying administrative requirements throughout their daily work (Definitive Healthcare and Vocera, 2019; Padden, 2019).

There have been many advocacy efforts to address nonessential policy barriers, but change was incremental until the federal government and many states removed barriers to care to respond to

---

[1] For background on this quote and those in other chapters, visit the NAM's Clinician Burnout Crisis in the Era of COVID-19: Insights from the Frontlines of Care webpage at: https://nam.edu/initiatives/clinician-resilience-and-well-being/clinician-burnout-crisis-in-the-era-of-covid-19/.

the COVID-19 public health emergency. This demonstrated that strategies to decrease health worker workload, which contributes to burnout, can be rapidly implemented on a wide scale. As a result of Centers for Medicare & Medicaid Services' emergency declaration blanket waivers, certain limitations to hiring out-of-state providers were lifted, documentation and reporting requirements were suspended or eliminated, and practice restrictions were modified—so that the health system could emphasize taking care of patients (CMS, 2020). To prepare for potential future emergencies, as COVID-19 becomes a more predictable and manageable threat, it will be important to understand the benefits that these flexibilities have had on the delivery of care and the health workforce, whether they should be sustained, and whether additional measures are needed. Fundamentally, health workers recognize what works in their local environments to execute a team-based model of care that meets patient needs and is positively linked to health worker well-being. A key way to maximize teamwork and efficiency in providing patient care is to fully leverage the training and education of all care team members (Smith et al., 2018). Organizational leaders should empower health workers to share their views, uncover barriers to team-based care, and work together with additional stakeholders such as funders and regulators to design a system that better serves the population and the health workforce.

Priority Area: Address compliance, regulatory, and policy barriers for daily work.

Goal 4.1.	Time spent on documentation is reduced to provide more time for meaningful professional activities and personal well-being.
Actors	Academic Institutions, Clinical Training Programs, and Accreditation Bodies
	Federal, State, and Local Governments
	Health Information Technology (IT) Companies
	Health Systems
	Health Workers
	Insurers and Payers
Actions	4.1.A. Revise policies and requirements for documentation that do not contribute to quality patient care.
	4.1.B. Remove low-value tasks from processes, rather than simply automating them.
	4.1.C. Measure time spent on documentation and set goals to reduce non-patient contact time.
	4.1.D. Use metrics to assess the nature and quality of workload in addition to achieving a reduction in overall time spent on administrative work.
	4.1.E. Include direct care workers in the refinement of electronic health records (EHRs) to ensure that proposed changes improve workflow.

Goal 4.2.	**Policies address hybrid, virtual, and in-person workflows to facilitate work-life integration and responsive patient care.**
Actors	Academic Institutions, Clinical Training Programs, and Accreditation Bodies
	Federal, State, and Local Governments
	Health Information Technology (IT) Companies
	Health Systems
	Health Workers
Actions	4.2.A. Institute paid leave and protections for health workers.
	4.2.B. Involve direct care workers in the development of hybrid workplace policies and provide training for teams to connect in-person and virtual workflows.
	4.2.C. Assess how virtual and in-person workflows connect and support each other.
	4.2.D. Fund infrastructure to support effective transitions to virtual or hybrid workflows for health workers.

Goal 4.3.	Prior authorization requirements are reimagined in a manner that places a focus on supporting quality patient care while also reducing unnecessary burden on health workers.
Actors	Academic Institutions, Clinical Training Programs, and Accreditation Bodies
	Federal, State, and Local Governments
	Health Information Technology (IT) Companies
	Health Systems
	Insurers and Payers
Actions	4.3.A. Eliminate prior authorization requirements if validated clinical decision support tools are used.
	4.3.B. Reduce the volume of prior authorizations needed and increase transparency of requirements.
	4.3.C. Standardize the prior authorization process with a single workflow so that payers can respond within fixed and defined timelines.
	4.3.D. Increase automation when appropriate and deploy health IT to ensure timely care for patients.
	4.3.E. Create rules and regulations that are general and as inclusive as possible. If exclusions are required, ensure they are limited and as specific as possible.

Goal 4.4.	Requirements are streamlined for health workers to comply with regulations and policies.
Actors	Academic Institutions, Clinical Training Programs, and Accreditation Bodies
	Federal, State, and Local Governments
	Health Information Technology (IT) Companies
	Health Systems
	Health Workers
	Insurers and Payers
	Private and Non-Profit Organizations
Actions	4.4.A. Form a public-private task force of experts, regulators, and health workers to identify frameworks and best practices for interpreting local-level rules and guidance that minimize burden.
	4.4.B. Standardize licensure processes, prepopulate necessary documents, and standardize timelines.
	4.4.C. Standardize facility and procedural credentialing with prepopulated documents, attestations, and other required paperwork.
	4.4.D. Re-evaluate mandatory learning and trainings to shorten or eliminate those that add to the administrative burden of health workers.

Goal 4.5.	Interstate practice is simplified and virtual services are easy for health workers and patients to use.
Actors	Academic Institutions, Clinical Training Programs, and Accreditation Bodies
	Federal, State, and Local Governments
	Health Information Technology (IT) Companies
	Health Systems
	Health Workers
	Insurers and Payers
Actions	4.5.A. Expand telehealth and virtual care for subsets of patients where such care has been shown to be safe and effective.
	4.5.B. Permanently remove certain licensure requirements to allow out-of-state health workers to perform telehealth services, and include telehealth credentialing and licensure within interstate compacts so that it is not an additional burden.
	4.5.C. Develop compensation models that facilitate asynchronous and continuous electronic messaging between the patient and the health care team.

NOTE: The list of actors in this table is not exhaustive. Many of the actors named in this table will need to plan and coordinate their actions with each other as part of a systems approach to health workforce well-being.

RELATED RESOURCES[2][1]

Conduct Workplace Assessment
- Tool: NASA Task Load Index (Agency for Healthcare Research and Quality)

---

[2] For additional resources, visit the NAM's Resource Compendium for Health Care Worker Well-Being webpage at: https://nam.edu/compendium-of-key-resources-for-improving-clinician-well-being/.

Enhance Workplace Efficiency
- Guide: Saving Time Playbook (American Medical Association)
- Calculator/Guide: Team Documentation: Improve Efficiency of EHR Documentation (Sinsky, 2014)
- Guide: Lean Health Care: Eliminate Waste and Spend Mre Time with Patients (Sinsky, 2015)

Examine Policies and Practices
- Guide: Debunking Regulatory Myths (American Medical Association)
- Guide: Getting Rid of Stupid Stuff: Reduce the Unnecessary Daily Burdens for Clinicians (Ashton, 2019)
- Framework: Putting Patients First by Reducing Administrative Tasks in Health Care (Erickson et al., 2017)
- Policy Considerations: Practice and Policy Reset Post-COVID-19: Reversion, Transition, or Transformation? (Sinsky and Linzer, 2020)
- Policy Action Items: 25x5 Symposium to Reduce Documentation Burden on U.S. Clinicians by 75% by 2025 Summary Report (Rossetti et al., 2021)
- Initiative: Occupational Therapy Licensure Compact (American Occupational Therapy Association)

5

Priority Area: Engage Effective Technology Tools

Optimize and expand the use of health information technologies that support health workers in providing high-quality patient care and serving population health, and minimize technologies that inhibit clinical decision-making or add to administrative burden.

> "The best redesign would be to really incorporate those who are working on the frontline in the decisions that are being made. Often the administration, who do not know what it's like to be swamped in the trenches of illness and disease, are the ones making the decisions." - Frontline Health Worker[1]

Well-designed health information technology (IT) can support the delivery and management of care and disease prevention, but poorly designed health IT can introduce frustration and errors into the care process, making it more difficult (NASEM, 2019). The implications can be pronounced in health care, where the ubiquity of electronic health records (EHRs) has significantly increased access to useful data for patient care and health care research. Unfortunately, EHRs are also among the most highly cited causes of health worker frustration and burnout (NASEM, 2019). Health workers report frustration stemming from several aspects of EHRs, including cumbersome design, decisions made at implementation (e.g., whether a nurse or medical assistant can document within fields

---

[1] For background on this quote and those in other chapters, visit the NAM's Clinician Burnout Crisis in the Era of COVID-19: Insights from the Frontlines of Care webpage at: https://nam.edu/initiatives/clinician-resilience-and-well-being/clinician-burnout-crisis-in-the-era-of-covid-19/.

outside of the chief complaint, what actions require an order, etc.), and unclear requirements from regulating bodies. EHRs also serve as the dataset for billing by health entities, with varying requirements and processes for reimbursement. Often, there are different data needs for what information must be recorded for the patient's health needs and what should be recorded for enhanced billing. In many instances, the lack of integration of administrative requirements in EHRs means the same note is duplicated by different team members, contributing to unnecessarily lengthy and unclear records. This tension can add to health worker stress and burnout (NASEM, 2019).

Inefficient workflows can be as or more problematic than the EHR for health workers. Interruptions and distractions "are associated with lower-quality and less safe care" (NASEM, 2019). They also "add to cognitive burden, delay task completion, and increase the risk of forgetting tasks" (NASEM, 2019). Health workers have suggested ways to deploy technologies—including but not limited to EHRs—to enable more efficient work and care and contact tracing in public health (Alotaibi and Federico, 2017; O'Shea, 2020). There are many opportunities to reorient health IT systems to reduce workplace stress and enhance professional well-being in the domains of design, implementation, and regulation. Health IT companies, via the EHR and other digital platforms, can have a tremendous effect on well-being if the private sector develops greater will to invest resources in well-designed health IT to serve all users, especially health workers.

Engage Effective Technology Tools | 45

Priority Area: Engage effective technology tools.	
Goal 5.1.	Health IT is user friendly and affordable, and meets standards co-designed with users.
Actors	Academic Institutions, Clinical Training Programs, and Accreditation Bodies
	Federal, State, and Local Governments
	Health Information Technology (IT) Companies
	Health Systems
	Health Workers
	Insurers and Payers
	Patients
	Private and Non-Profit Organizations
Actions	5.1.A. Promote necessary interactions of stakeholders to design and improve documentation systems and leverage better technology solutions that are health-oriented and human-centered.
	5.1.B. Conduct research on how to develop and apply health IT that supports health workers in care delivery, including prevention services and contact tracing.
	5.1.C. Define standards for all health technologies to be clinically useful and accurate. Include standards for the following domains: usability/user experience before and after implementation of technology, degree of cognitive load, and degree of clinical decision-making support.
	5.1.D. Create market advantages for producing technologies that are human-centered and highly user friendly.

Goal 5.2.	Health IT is interoperable across disciplines and platforms to enhance team-based care and continuity of care.
Actors	Academic Institutions, Clinical Training Programs, and Accreditation Bodies
	Federal, State, and Local Governments
	Health Information Technology (IT) Companies
	Health Systems
	Health Workers
	Patients
Actions	5.2.A. Encourage the adoption of existing interoperability standards and the development of enhanced interoperability standards.
	5.2.B. Discourage proprietary solutions that are not interoperable.

Goal 5.3.	Technology innovations improve both patient care and workload of health workers.
Actors	Federal, State, and Local Governments
	Health Information Technology (IT) Companies
	Health Systems
	Health Workers
	Patients
	Professional and Specialty Societies
Actions	5.3.A. Deploy health IT using human-centered design and human factors and systems engineering approaches to ensure the effectiveness, efficiency, usability, and safety of the technology.
	5.3.B. Develop widgets that focus on documenting individual services.
	5.3.C. Establish a joint public-private fund for technology and EHR optimization to improve workloads and workflows.
	5.3.D. Establish partnerships with social service agencies to connect patients to services and ensure their pertinent health information can be shared in a meaningful way.

Goal 5.4.	Technologies facilitate increased personal connections with patients.
Actors	Health Information Technology (IT) Companies
	Health Systems
	Health Workers
	Patients
Actions	5.4.A. Automate processes to streamline the health care team's workflow (e.g., ambient artificial intelligence, virtual scribes, or voice assistants) to allow health workers to focus on listening to patients, rather than manually documenting notes at the computer, and increase patient safety.
	5.4.B. Offload and/or automate the administrative tracking tasks associated with preventive care (e.g., natural language processing technologies for inbox management), so health workers can focus on more complex care needs and communicating information to the patient.

Goal 5.5.	The use of technology is understood and established as an enabler to streamline care.
Actors	Academic Institutions, Clinical Training Programs, and Accreditation Bodies
	Health Information Technology (IT) Companies
	Health Systems
	Health Workers
	Insurers and Payers
	Patients
Actions	5.5.A. Employ technology tools to maintain personal safety (e.g., ability to videoconference into a patient's room when appropriate) when treating communicable diseases or while calling on other experts and members of the care team (e.g., virtual reality headsets).
	5.5.B. Use EHR audit-log data to characterize the work environment and assess whether interventions to improve the environment were effective.
	5.5.C. Create publicly available accountability measures.
	5.5.D. Examine the benefits and drawbacks to using technology, video, and phone consultations in addressing workforce burnout and patient health.

NOTE: The list of actors in this table is not exhaustive. Many of the actors named in this table will need to plan and coordinate their actions with each other as part of a systems approach to health workforce well-being.

RELATED RESOURCES[2]

<u>Enhance Workplace Efficiency</u>
- Calculator/Guide: Team Documentation: Improve Efficiency of EHR Documentation (Sinsky, 2014)
- Guide: Taming the Electronic Health Record Playbook (Jin et al., 2022)
- Case Study: HCA Healthcare's Program to Streamline Documentation for Nursing (American Hospital Association)
- Case Study: Just in Time: EHR Training at Atlantic Medical Group (American Hospital Association)
- Commentary: Evaluating and Reducing Cognitive Load Should Be a Priority for Machine Learning (Ehrmann et al., 2022)
- Framework: Trusted Exchange Framework and Common Agreement (Office of the National Coordinator for Health Information Technology)

<u>Strengthen Leadership Behaviors</u>
- Webinar: Integrating Patient Safety and Clinician Wellbeing (Privitera and MacNamee, 2021)

---

[2] For additional resources, visit the NAM's Resource Compendium for Health Care Worker Well-Being webpage at: https://nam.edu/compendium-of-key-resources-for-improving-clinician-well-being/.

6

Priority Area: Institutionalize Well-Being as a Long-Term Value

Ensure COVID-19 recovery efforts address the toll on health worker well-being now and in the future, and bolster the public health and health care systems for future emergencies.

> "I felt forgotten about by upper-level hospital management, family, friends, neighbors, etc. This affected my personal mental health because I felt like I was fighting this invisible war every day, watching people die all the time, dealing with a very sick patient whose family doesn't believe COVID is real."
> - Frontline Health Worker[1]

Health care teams and public health workers experienced extraordinary fear, fatigue, isolation, and moral distress and injury during COVID-19, and recommendations for resilience often place the onus on the individual rather than the system. The nation must acknowledge that the health workforce will require recovery from the trauma of the pandemic, and that stress and distress are long-term issues that must be addressed with longitudinal, long-term solutions. In addition, the health care delivery system will face other challenges after the pandemic, including the demand for delayed and deferred care for non-COVID-19 patients, as well as emerging long-term side effects of COVID-19 for patients and health workers. The public health response to the pandemic may continue for

---
[1] For background on this quote and those in other chapters, visit the NAM's Clinician Burnout Crisis in the Era of COVID-19: Insights from the Frontlines of Care webpage at: https://nam.edu/initiatives/clinician-resilience-and-well-being/clinician-burnout-crisis-in-the-era-of-covid-19/.

years via surveillance programs, contact tracing, and other monitoring and evaluation efforts.

Understanding that burnout among health workers was a significant challenge prior to COVID-19, and the extent of the traumatic stress and injury from this period is yet to be determined, it is essential that well-being is institutionalized as a key priority at all levels of the health system. Furthermore, policies and protocols should reflect the dynamic nature of responses and prioritize health worker well-being. At the organizational level, leaders and health workers need to understand that health worker well-being is essential for safe, high-quality patient care. Leaders should use a systems approach for appropriate work system redesign and implementation, and health workers must be equipped with the required commitment, infrastructure, resources, accountability frameworks, and culture that supports well-being.

As seen during the pandemic, an underfunded public health system, including federal agencies and local, regional, and state health departments, has negative implications for the health of people across the country (Farberman et al., 2020). It is important that public health and health care systems guard against "active forgetting," emphasize lessons learned from the pandemic, and address emerging questions on how the nation might prepare for the next pandemic or national emergency. Investing in infrastructure and institutionalizing well-being as a value are long-term approaches to growing a culture that provides the health workforce with the necessary supports to recover from the trauma of serving during the pandemic, and to bolstering a system committed to supporting well-being for the long-term.

Priority Area: Institutionalize well-being as a long-term value.		
Goal 6.1.	Health worker and learner well-being are prioritized, reflected in, and operationalized in strategic plans and core values.	
Actors		Academic Institutions, Clinical Training Programs, and Accreditation Bodies
		Federal, State, and Local Governments
		Health Information Technology (IT) Companies
		Health Systems
		Health Workers
		Insurers and Payers
		Professional and Specialty Societies
Actions	6.1.A. Define the organization's ideal future state, guided by a culture that institutionalizes well-being as a core value.	
	6.1.B. Communicate that health worker well-being is essential for safe, high-quality patient care.	
	6.1.C. Commit to infrastructure, resources, accountability, and a culture that supports well-being.	
	6.1.D. Ensure a systems approach for appropriate work system redesign and implementation.	
	6.1.E. Provide training for health workers and learners that offers interactive, engaging formats that build communication and collaboration and goes beyond mandatory e-learning.	
	6.1.F. Provide coverage and compensation for direct care workers to engage in meetings and other decision-making forums.	
	6.1.G. Develop hybrid work policies to enable health workers to complete their work from home.	
	6.1.H. Plan for sufficient reserves of personal protective equipment (PPE) and other resources in preparation for future emergencies.	

Goal 6.2.	The effects of COVID-19 on the well-being of the health workforce are addressed.
Actors	Federal, State, and Local Governments
	Health Systems
	Health Workers
	Insurers and Payers
	Private and Non-Profit Organizations
	Professional and Specialty Societies
Actions	6.2.A. Appropriate funds for the National Health Workforce commission (authorized as part of the Affordable Care Act) to gather real-time workforce data.
	6.2.B. Secure long-term funding to treat and support those who experience acute physical and mental stress and long-term effects from providing care in response to COVID-19.
	6.2.C. Facilitate adequate time off and provide mental health resources without stigma or punishment.
	6.2.D. Establish a national platform or network that can rapidly share, implement, and test models or solutions for transitioning from acute COVID-19 care to institutionalizing long-term well-being.
	6.2.E. Streamline the discharge planning Condition of Participation (focusing on the most pertinent information to discharge patients to post-acute facilities), in recognition of health workforce shortages and administrative flexibilities allowed during COVID-19.
	6.2.F. Grant relief on timeframes related to pre- and post-admission patient assessments and evaluation criteria-both to ensure patients are treated in a timely manner and to allow health care settings and health workers to better manage an influx of non-COVID-19 patients returning for care, in recognition of health workforce shortages and administrative flexibilities allowed during COVID-19.

Institutionalize Well-Being as a Long-Term Value | 55

Goal 6.3.	A strong and coordinated national public health infrastructure has a thriving public health workforce.
Actors	Academic Institutions, Clinical Training Programs, and Accreditation Bodies
	Federal, State, and Local Governments
	Health Systems
Actions	6.3.A. Invest in cross-cutting foundational public health capabilities, including threats assessment and monitoring, all-hazards preparedness, public communication and education, community partnership development, and program management and leadership.
	6.3.B. Re-invest in the public health workforce through training and education opportunities.
	6.3.C. Modernize surveillance and data systems.
	6.3.D. Provide full-year funding for federal agencies that is not disease-specific.
	6.3.E. Increase investment in the U.S. Department of Health and Human Services (HHS) Prevention and Public Health Fund (authorized as part of the Affordable Care Act).
	6.3.F. Increase funding for the Centers for Disease Control and Prevention (CDC) community health emergency preparedness programs.
	6.3.G. Use available data and science to inform decisions, priorities, and policies.

NOTE: The list of actors in this table is not exhaustive. Many of the actors named in this table will need to plan and coordinate their actions with each other as part of a systems approach to health workforce well-being.

RELATED RESOURCES[2][1]

Cultivate a Culture of Connection and Support
- Guide: Conversation and Action Guide to Support Staff Well-Being and Joy in Work during and After the COVID-19 Pandemic (Institute for Healthcare Improvement)
- Guide: Well-Being Playbook 2.0: A COVID-19 Resource for Hospital and Health System Leaders (American Hospital Association)
- Guide: Building Bridges Between Practicing Physicians and Administrators: Improve Physician-Administrator Relationships and Enhance Engagement (DeChant, 2021)
- Organizational Best Practices: At the Heart of the Pandemic: Nursing Peer Support (Godfrey and Scott, 2021)
- Organizational Graphic: Psychological PPE: Promote Health Care Workforce Mental Health and Well-Being (Institute for Healthcare Improvement)
- Overview of COVID-19 Resources by Roles: COVID-19: Stress and Coping Resources (American Hospital Association)

Advance Organizational Commitment
- Guide: A Guide to Promoting Health Care Workforce Well-Being During and After the Pandemic (Institute for Healthcare Improvement)
- Guide: Creating the Organizational Foundation for Joy in Medicine: Organizational Changes Lead to Physician Satisfaction (Sinsky et al., 2017)
- Guide: Wellness with COVID: Contagious Strategies to Promote Pharmacy Well-Being (American Society of Health-System Pharmacists)
- Brief: A Call to Action: Improving Clinician Well-Being and Patient Care and Safety (Schmidt and Aly, 2020)
- Discussion Paper/Guide: Healing the Professional Culture of Medicine (Shanafelt et al., 2019)
- Fact Sheet: Prevention and Public Health Fund Fact Sheet (American Public Health Association)

---

[2] For additional resources, visit the NAM's Resource Compendium for Health Care Worker Well-Being webpage at: https://nam.edu/compendium-of-key-resources-for-improving-clinician-well-being/.

Strengthen Leadership Behaviors

- Compilation: Leading Through Crisis: A Resource Compendium for Nurse Leaders (American Organization for Nursing Leadership)
- Guide: Well-Being Playbook: A Guide for Hospital and Health System Leaders (American Hospital Association)
- Guide: Appreciative Inquiry Principles: Ask "What Went Well" to Foster Positive Organizational Culture (Frankel and Beyt, 2016)
- Guide: Cultivating Leadership: Measure and Assess Leader Behaviors to Improve Professional Well-Being (Swenson and Shanafelt, 2020)
- Strategies: Executive Leadership and Physician Well-Being: Nine Organizational Strategies to Promote Engagement and Reduce Burnout (Shanafelt and Noseworthy, 2017)
- Discussion Paper: A Call to Action: Align Well-Being and Antiracism Strategies (Barrett et al., 2021)
- Guide: Grief Leadership: Leadership in the Wake of Tragedy (Uniformed Services University)

7

Priority Area: Recruit and Retain a Diverse and Inclusive Health Workforce

Promote careers in the health professions and increase pathways and systems for a diverse, inclusive, and thriving workforce.

"The energy of caring for the sickest of the sick and the collaboration between all physicians and nurses/staff was uplifting and life affirming in the darkest of times."
- Frontline Health Worker[1]

Health care and public health workers were lauded as heroes early in the COVID-19 pandemic, as they operated under high-pressure circumstances and navigated disease uncertainties. However, stress, burnout, and mental health challenges experienced by frontline workers have accelerated departures from direct patient care and disease prevention and monitoring across the country. As mentioned earlier, the emotional well-being of clinicians of color was also disproportionately impacted during COVID-19, as they experienced heightened discrimination and harassment. National media highlighted unacceptable working conditions for health workers; concerns for the safety of the patients in their care due to persistent staffing shortages; and in many cases, the inability to work and advise at the top of their training and education as health care and public health specialists (Yong, 2021). Cultivating multidisciplinary team-based care is important not only to efficiently

---

[1] For background on this quote and those in other chapters, visit the NAM's Clinician Burnout Crisis in the Era of COVID-19: Insights from the Frontlines of Care webpage at: https://nam.edu/initiatives/clinician-resilience-and-well-being/clinician-burnout-crisis-in-the-era-of-covid-19/.

and effectively navigate the complexities of the U.S. health care delivery system, but also to support health workers in providing safe patient care and increasing their overall well-being (Sinsky et al., 2020; Smith et al., 2018). Health systems should fully leverage the education, certifications, and experiences of all care team members, fostering a clinical care environment of mutual professional respect (Smith et al., 2018).

The nation must acknowledge that a functioning U.S. health system requires ongoing care for and investment in health workers. Demonstrating the importance of the health workforce includes prioritizing retention of the existing skilled workforce, investing in continuing education, and restoring a sense of inclusion and meaning in health care and public health education and training. If the goals described in earlier chapters are not achieved, positive work and learning environments are not cultivated, barriers to daily work are not removed, and well-being is not institutionalized as a long-term value, many applicants and potential future health professionals may be discouraged from pursuing or maintaining these careers–to the detriment of the nation's health.

Furthermore, it is paramount to promote careers in the health professions to build a strong health workforce that reflects a growing, aging, and more racially and ethnically diverse U.S. population, while also actively advancing health equity. The historical and continued lack of diversity and inclusion in the health workforce, which overtly and covertly reinforces exclusion of people of color, people who are LGBTQIA+ (lesbian, gay, bisexual, transgender, queer/questioning, intersex, and ally/asexual), people with disabilities, and other underrepresented groups in the health professions, is another structural barrier to recruiting and retaining a diverse and inclusive workforce. Although unprecedented surges in medical and public health school applications were reported in 2021, it is unclear how they have affected enrollment in training programs, and workforce shortages remain. The shortages are especially acute among professions such as aides, assistants, and nurses (e.g., a shortage of more than 1 million nurses is expected). In regions where shortages are chronic, such as rural areas where access to health care is limited, the recruitment of health workers is uniquely challenging (Bhatnagar et al., 2022; Pollack, 2022). Admissions offices speculate this application surge is partly because COVID-19 accelerated people's motivations to join the pandemic response and help alleviate social injustices (Boyle, 2021; Warnick, 2021).

In response, educational systems must adequately scale to meet the demands of incoming students and ensure there are enough placements, embracing cohorts that are more diverse than any before 2021 through equitable and holistic admissions processes and cultural humility practices (Boyle, 2021). Insufficient numbers of nurse faculty and clinical placements continue to severely limit the capacities of nursing schools to accept all qualified applicants and train future practitioners (NASEM, 2021). While training new health professionals takes time, efforts to advance team-based care can help address workforce shortages in the near-term through the benefits of well-being for high-functioning teams and improved patient care (Smith et al., 2018).

Caring for others is a noble calling, and health care and public health roles offer numerous opportunities for intellectual gratification and interactions with people from all facets of life. Society needs to address the challenges and leverage lessons learned during the pandemic to commit to improving the health system, so health workers and patients flourish. It does not matter if resilience is instilled in individual future health workers if they enter systems that diminish their abilities to thrive (NAM, 2022).

Priority Area: Recruit and retain a diverse and inclusive health workforce.	
Goal 7.1.	The size and composition of the health workforce reflects the demand and diversity of the U.S. population.
Actors	Academic Institutions, Clinical Training Programs, and Accreditation Bodies
	Federal, State, and Local Governments
	Health Systems
Actions	7.1.A. Train, hire, and retain people from underrepresented and marginalized communities in health care and public health (see actions to support diverse, equitable, accessible, and inclusive settings in Chapter 1).
	7.1.B. Provide debt relief opportunities for students and workers through employer programs and expanded eligibility for loan forgiveness.
	7.1.C. Invest in educational pathways and programs such as: • pipeline programs and partnerships among high schools, technical schools, and universities to allow emergency medical technicians, certified nursing assistants, and armed forces medics to apply work hours toward clinical professions; • targeted scholarships or tuition support for nursing students or nursing educators to increase workforce numbers; and • onsite graduate school and professional development programs to retain experienced nurses.
	7.1.D. Allow extensions to residency cap-building periods for new graduate medical education programs to address recruitment, resource availability, and program operations.
	7.1.E. Fund graduate nurse education programs to address significant worker shortages across the health system.
	7.1.F. Expand and scale support for a national Reserve Nurse Training Corps using the military's Reserve Officers' Training Corps as a model, including undergraduate tuition payment and service commitment.
	7.1.G. Leverage the role of the U.S. Surgeon General to prioritize and communicate the significance of addressing health workforce well-being.

Goal 7.2.	The health system retains health workers who have personal caregiving responsibilities.
Actors	Academic Institutions, Clinical Training Programs, and Accreditation Bodies
	Federal, State, and Local Governments
	Health Systems
	Private and Non-Profit Organizations
Actions	7.2.A. Revise policies to offer flexibility for clinical schedules, job-sharing, remote work, and opportunities to re-enter the workforce.
	7.2.B. Increase the duration of and pay for parental leave.
	7.2.C. Invest in and improve childcare opportunities.
	7.2.D. Increase diversity in leadership, management, and health care teams.
	7.2.E. Review compensation to ensure equitable practices across the organization.

Goal 7.3.	**Health care environments are person-centered and safe for health workers.**
Actors	Academic Institutions, Clinical Training Programs, and Accreditation Bodies
	Federal, State, and Local Governments
	Health Systems
	Health Workers
	Private and Non-Profit Organizations
Actions	7.3.A. Establish and follow staffing plans that reflect effective team composition and balanced workloads to provide safe patient care.
	7.3.B. Create clear criteria for the appropriate use of mandatory overtime to ensure it is applied only in emergency circumstances.
	7.3.C. Fund testing and implementation of interventions that improve occupational safety for health workers.

Recruit and Retain a Diverse and Inclusive Health Workforce | 65

Goal 7.4.	Health workers have the infrastructure to support their work to improve population health.
Actors	Federal, State, and Local Governments
	Health Systems
	Health Workers
	Insurers and Payers
	Patients
Actions	7.4.A. Incentivize payers to invest in providing quality community resources to address barriers that patients face in obtaining care and attaining their full health potential (the social determinants of health [SDOH]).
	7.4.B. Provide greater flexibility for Medicare Advantage to reimburse health workers for addressing SDOH.
	7.4.C. Explore the integration of SDOH as a factor in payment policy and the infrastructure needed to support connections to social services. Elements include: • incorporating standardized SDOH billing codes into health worker IT systems, such as electronic health records (EHRs) and care management platforms; • aligning incentives for senior and frontline leaders to address SDOH for patients and populations; and • recognizing and rewarding health workers for addressing SDOH.

Goal 7.5.	Health workers and learners are inspired and equipped to meet the challenges of caring for the nation.
Actors	Academic Institutions, Clinical Training Programs, and Accreditation Bodies
	Federal, State, and Local Governments
	Health Systems
	Health Workers
	Media and Communications
	Professional and Specialty Societies
Actions	7.5.A. Each profession creates a future vision of what it means to fulfill their duties.
	7.5.B. Create incentives to facilitate team-based care.
	7.5.C. Administer surveys to students pre-matriculation through graduation to assess and respond in a timely manner to personal and professional experiences along the educational pathway.
	7.5.D. Invest in continuing education.
	7.5.E. Develop health worker reserves to address emergent needs and large-scale disasters.
	7.5.F. Conduct message testing and communications research to develop media campaigns that highlight the joy and fulfillment of the health professions, as well as health worker contributions during the COVID-19 pandemic.
	7.5.G. Launch a campaign with influential voices in health that targets multiple sectors of society.

NOTE: The list of actors in this table is not exhaustive. Many of the actors named in this table will need to plan and coordinate their actions with each other as part of a systems approach to health workforce well-being.

RELATED RESOURCES[2][1]

<u>Examine Policies and Practices</u>
- Strategies: Policy Strategies for Addressing Current Threats to the U.S. Nursing Workforce (Costa and Friese, 2022)
- Survey: Matriculating Student Questionnaire (Association of American Medical Colleges)

<u>Strengthen Leadership Behaviors</u>
- Discussion Paper/Action Items: Physician Well-Being 2.0: Where We Are and Where We Are Going (Shanafelt, 2021)
- Discussion Paper/Action Items: Getting Through COVID-19: Keeping Clinicians in the Workforce (Barrett et al., 2021a)
- Discussion Paper: A Call to Action: Align Well-Being and Antiracism Strategies (Barrett et al., 2021b)

---

[2] For additional resources, visit the NAM's Resource Compendium for Health Care Worker Well-Being webpage at: https://nam.edu/compendium-of-key-resources-for-improving-clinician-well-being/.

Summary and Conclusion

No single actor is responsible for making the significant investments needed to ensure sustainable, system-wide changes and to achieve the vision set out in this National Plan. Investment in health worker well-being must come from multiple levels. These actions must include individual health systems and training programs—both large and small—committing to a baseline understanding of burnout and distress in their workforce. Then, interventions must be implemented with frontline health workers that include public and private payers streamlining processes and requirements, providing reimbursements for mental health care, and supporting efforts to enhance well-being; developers of health IT improving EHRs and innovating to be more human-centered; and federal and state governments investing in wide scale research, as well as tracking and removing barriers to allow funding to flow to work and learning environments.

The goals, actions, and actors identified in this National Plan are interconnected and aim to support health worker well-being and a thriving U.S. health system. Improving health worker well-being is a shared responsibility that requires collective action by all actors in the U.S. health system and those who influence the systems that support health. Health leaders play an important role in their institutions and must work together with frontline health workers to address barriers to well-being. Community members, from patients to the public, private and non-profit institutions to media organizations, are also called upon to join this burgeoning social movement for health worker well-being and start spreading change on a massive scale.

Leaders of health, public health, and educational institutions must understand the extent and drivers of workplace stress and burnout at the organizational level. Frontline health workers and learners are vital partners for implementing context-specific interventions that will create safe and supportive work and learning environments. Our health workers and learners cannot be expected to work in violent, threatening, and unsafe conditions, or be made to feel unwelcome in environments that are not diverse, equitable, inclusive, and accessible. As a nation, we must understand the effects of COVID-19 and public health crises on the well-being of the health workforce, protect their mental health, and reduce the stigma associated with speaking about these issues now and in the future.

At the national level, policies, payment structures, and other key systems governing care and disease prevention must align to focus on human connection and trust in health care. We must review and revise our technology, rules, regulations, and policies to streamline care and reduce the burden in service of the critical health worker-patient relationship. We must institutionalize well-being as a value to ensure the health and longevity of those who care for us and train, hire, and retain a health workforce that reflects the diversity of the U.S. population.

Much like how the national movement to improve the safety and quality of care delivery has gained ground over the last 20 years, improving health worker well-being will be a long journey. While there is no finish line, every step makes a difference in improving the environment for our health workforce and brings us closer to experiencing a health system where both health workers and patients thrive.

How will the nation know we are on the right path? Key indicators of progress are more health systems using validated surveys to track health worker well-being and burnout, and training programs that integrate health worker well-being into their strategic plans and educational curricula. Other signs of positive change at the national level include increased funding streams and evidence-based policy making that support health workforce well-being, and the design, deployment, and accessibility of human-centered technologies that increase the efficiency and safety of the health workforce and simultaneously enhance patient care.

Where do we go from here? An ecosystem of actors that work collectively to coordinate, facilitate, report, and enable accountability will be necessary for long-term change. A coalition should catalyze action across professions, settings, and regions; fairly represent all health professions; and unequivocally embrace the principles of diversity, equity, inclusion, and accessibility. With this National Plan, the key elements to create a social movement for health workforce well-being in the United States are identified, and we must seize this COVID-19 crisis as a window of opportunity (see Chapter 1). Next will be a focus on the voices of newly committed and re-committed actors to spark widespread change, advocacy of the actions outlined in this National Plan, and mass communication efforts to amplify the messages of this National Plan.

This moment demands urgency. Challenges to health worker well-being were documented prior to the pandemic, and COVID-19 has only deepened these issues and led to a health workforce that is too small and has high levels of burnout and distress. We cannot witness and not act, as our health workers continuing to sound the alarm for reprieve from the multitude of stressors that have strained and drained our health workforce. Immediate and sustained action to address health worker burnout and improve well-being is imperative to ensure that the United States has a health workforce that can support our population now and in the future. While we have made progress, more commitment and investment are necessary for sustainable change. Improving health worker well-being is a societal issue—it is our ethical obligation to take action to protect those who care for all of us.

APPENDIX A

Background on the Clinician Well-Being Collaborative and National Plan Process

Established in 2017, the National Academy of Medicine (NAM) Action Collaborative on Clinician Well-Being and Resilience (the Collaborative) has made important contributions to address the burnout crisis by aligning over 100 key players within the U.S. health system and galvanizing a growing network of more than 200 organizations committed to reversing trends in clinician burnout. The Collaborative has made great strides in raising the visibility of clinician anxiety, burnout, depression, stress, and suicide, as well as improving baseline understanding of challenges to clinician well-being. The Collaborative also continues to advance evidence-based, multidisciplinary solutions to improve patient care by caring for the caregiver.

PHASE I (2017 TO 2020): BUILDING A COMMUNITY AROUND CLINICIAN WELL-BEING

At the outset, the Collaborative focused on creating a community for stakeholders to discuss clinician well-being and share ideas. Working groups identified evidence-based strategies to engage leadership, break the culture of silence, organize promising practices and metrics, address workload and workflow, and act on recommendations to improve clinician well-being. Products and activities of the Collaborative include an online knowledge hub, a series of NAM Perspectives papers, an art exhibit, and a conceptual model that reflects the domains affecting clinician well-being (all materials listed are available at: https://nam.edu/initiatives/clinician-resilience-and-well-being/).

PHASE II (2021 TO 2022): CREATING A NATIONAL PLAN FOR HEALTH WORKFORCE WELL-BEING

Informed by discussions with multidisciplinary experts and stakeholders during COVID-19, the Collaborative reflected on how to capitalize on the lessons learned and opportunities to strengthen workforce well-being. Since 2021, the Collaborative has been organized into three Working Groups:

1. The Working Group on Implementing Tools to Improve Clinician Well-Being aims to catalyze the uptake of evidence-based practices and the implementation of tools to support health care leaders in improving clinician well-being on the frontlines of care.
2. The Working Group on Mobilizing National Stakeholders for Clinician Well-Being aims to create a national strategy for clinician well-being by mobilizing and sustaining the engagement, resources, and accountability of key health care stakeholders.
3. The Working Group on Navigating the Impacts of COVID-19 on Clinician Well-Being aims to support the health care workforce during the pandemic and to apply emerging lessons from COVID-19.

In November 2021, members of the Collaborative's Steering Committee met to identify priority areas to advance health care worker well-being. The Steering Committee participated in six meetings between December 2021 and May 2022 to lead the conceptualization, outlining, drafting, and editing of the National Plan, with input from all Collaborative members. A draft of the National Plan was made publicly available for any member of the public to provide feedback in May 2022. The final text of the National Plan is the culmination of committee deliberations, consideration of public input, and completion of the NAM peer review process.

APPENDIX B

Background from the National Academies Consensus Study Report and Other Reference Materials for the National Plan's Priority Areas

The foundation for the National Plan's priority areas was the goals and recommendations from the consensus study report Taking Action Against Clinician Burnout: A Systems Approach to Professional Well-Being[1], and the activities and products of the Collaborative's Working Groups, including:

1. Working Group on Implementing Tools to Improve Clinician Well-Being,
2. Working Group on Mobilizing National Stakeholders for Clinician Well-Being, and
3. Working Group on Navigating the Impacts of COVID-19 on Clinician Well-Being.

CONSENSUS STUDY REPORT GOALS FOR REDUCING CLINICIAN BURNOUT AND ENHANCING PROFESSIONAL WELL-BEING[2]

1. "Create Positive Work Environments: Transform health care work systems by creating positive work environments that

---

[1] https://doi.org/10.17226/25521.
[2] For more information, see: National Academies of Sciences, Engineering, and Medicine. 2019. Taking Action Against Clinician Burnout: A Systems Approach to Professional Well-Being. Washington, DC: The National Academies Press. https://doi.org/10.17226/25521.

prevent and reduce burnout, foster professional well-being, and support quality care.
2. **Create Positive Learning Environments:** Transform health professions education and training to optimize learning environments that prevent and reduce burnout and foster professional well-being.
3. **Reduce Administrative Burden:** Prevent and reduce the negative consequences on clinicians' professional well-being that result from laws, regulations, policies, and standards promulgated by health care policy, regulatory, and standards-setting entities, including government agencies (federal, state, and local), professional organizations, and accreditors.
4. **Enable Technology Solutions:** Optimize the use of health information technologies to support clinicians in providing high-quality patient care.
5. **Provide Support to Clinicians and Learners:** Reduce the stigma and eliminate the barriers associated with obtaining the support and services needed to prevent and alleviate burnout symptoms, facilitate recovery from burnout, and foster professional well-being among learners and practicing clinicians.
6. **Invest in Research:** Provide dedicated funding for research on clinician professional well-being."

WORKING GROUP ON IMPLEMENTING TOOLS TO IMPROVE CLINICIAN WELL-BEING

To help health systems take action, the NAM Resource Compendium for Health Care Worker Well-Being[3] organizes available strategies and tools into six essential elements for health worker well-being:

1. **Advance Organizational Commitment:** Organizational commitment involves visible actions and investments to show that a systematic approach to decreasing health care worker burnout and improving well-being is being undertaken.
2. **Strengthen Leadership Behaviors:** Leadership must believe in the importance of health care worker well-being, commit

---
[3] https://nam.edu/compendium-of-key-resources-for-improving-clinician-well-being/.

to making well-being a strategic priority, and support a culture of well-being. Leadership at all levels is important, as are tools for accountability.
3. Conduct Workplace Assessment: Measurement is essential to understanding the extent and severity of burnout and the well-being of the members of any workforce, and to determining the effectiveness of intervention strategies.
4. Examine Policies and Practices: Health care workers experience moral distress and injury when the policies and practices of their organization conflict with their professional commitment to patient care and their ability to do their work. A resilient organization will periodically reassess its policies and practices and eliminate those that are no longer relevant or no longer required.
5. Enhance Workplace Efficiency: Workplace efficiency embodies practices that are geared toward facilitating and streamlining staff duties while maintaining clinical excellence.
6. Cultivate a Culture of Connection and Support: An organization can best support its health care workforce by giving people the ability to do their jobs and then allowing them to return safely home with time and emotional energy to engage in their personal lives with their family, friends, and community.

WORKING GROUP ON MOBILIZING NATIONAL STAKEHOLDERS FOR CLINICIAN WELL-BEING

Convening on Reducing Documentation and Administrative Burden (January 31, 2022)

More information is available at: https://nam.edu/event/reducing-documentation-administrative-burden-for-clinician-well-being/.

Meeting Objectives:

The Centers for Medicare & Medicaid Services (CMS) and American Medical Association (AMA) collaborated on revisions to the Evaluation and Management (E/M) office visit Current Procedural Terminology (CPT) codes that became effective In January 2021. These changes were intended to address documentation standards that cause administrative burden among health care workers in nearly every specialty.

The overarching objective of this meeting was to take the principles of implementing the E/M CPT code changes and documentation-related administrative burden and apply them to the broader concept of putting policy change into action. The NAM Clinician Well-Being Collaborative intended to assemble policy and health care stakeholders to:

1. Discuss successes and challenges in operationalizing documentation policy change,
2. Examine the impact of these specific coding revisions on administrative burden, and
3. Identify opportunities to inform the process of policy change on a broader scale.

Meeting participants generated lessons learned from the E/M CPT code changes to guide the formulation, implementation, and assessment of future administrative relief policies that will have positive, interprofessional effects on clinician well-being.

Convening on Health Technology for Reducing Burden
(April 8, 2022)

More information is available at: https://nam.edu/event/health-technology-to-reduce-burnout/.

Meeting Objectives:

Technology can be both a source of and solution to the challenges of prior authorization, in-basket management, credentialing, documentation burden, and other major drivers of clinician burnout. The NAM Clinician Well-Being Collaborative assembled industry leaders, policy makers, and clinician stakeholders to spotlight promising technologies that alleviate provider burden and enhance patient-centered care, then explored key opportunities for deploying technologies at the health care organization level on a national scale.

The virtual public convening:
1. Highlighted innovations with promise for rapid implementation and broad scale that are available now, noted the persistent barriers to penetrating real-world small and large practice settings to be resolved, and identified forward-looking technologies to reduce provider burden.
2. Examined data that illustrate technology-related pain points for frontline care providers and that serve as opportunities for innovation.
3. Learned from implementers who have successfully deployed technologies at their institutions to reduce provider burden and can spotlight technologies in development in a variety of practice settings.
4. Discussed the role of federal barriers and incentives in catalyzing implementation of technology innovations to reduce provider burden on a national scale.

Convening on Leveraging the Role of Payers and Regulators in the Health Worker Well-Being Movement
(October 3, 2022)

More information is available at: https://nam.edu/event/leveraging-the-role-of-payers-and-regulators-in-the-health-worker-well-being-movement/.

Meeting Objectives:
The NAM Clinician Well-Being Collaborative assembled Collaborative members who are industry leaders and clinician stakeholders, as well as regulators and payers in the private and public sector, for a closed discussion on the structural impacts of the current payment system on burnout and moral injury in order to envision a future care delivery system that can enhance health worker well-being.

The convening:
1. Examined elements of the current payment system that create barriers to health worker well-being.
2. Highlighted the role of payers and regulators in alleviating health worker burnout and distress.

3. Discussed pathways forward for payers and regulators to promote health worker well-being.

WORKING GROUP ON NAVIGATING THE IMPACTS OF COVID-19 ON CLINICIAN WELL-BEING

Convening on Clinician Retention in the Era of COVID: Uniting the Health Workforce to Optimize Well-Being (March 15, 2022)

More information is available at: https://nam.edu/event/clinician-retention-in-the-era-of-covid-uniting-the-health-workforce-to-optimize-well-being/.

Meeting Objectives:

The COVID-19 pandemic has brought clinician well-being to the forefront of national attention. Staffing shortages have exacerbated an already thinly stretched health care workforce that is also experiencing violence and harassment in the workplace and significant moral injury. In addition to addressing the acute challenges of COVID-19, embedding well-being as a value is foundational for health care organizations to address the systemic barriers to clinician well-being and create environments that support clinician retention and expertise in patient care. Therefore, we need to unite in our journey to strengthen well-being with and for the health care workforce.

The NAM's Action Collaborative on Clinician Well-Being and Resilience assembled industry leaders, C-Suite members, and frontline health care workers to share perspectives on challenges and barriers, pinpoint solutions, and discuss actionable strategies to mitigate burnout and strengthen the health care workforce. The public meeting highlighted:

- Individual-level stressors in the context of COVID-19,
- Institutional-level challenges and opportunities to support workforce well-being, and
- National-level levers for improving workforce well-being, the pipeline of health workers, and stemming the shortage.

The meeting featured lessons from three institutions about their journeys in creating wellness action plans for and with their front-line staff with the intention to encourage other health-serving institutions to begin or continue their journeys.

APPENDIX C

References

DEFINITIONS

American Medical Association (AMA). 2020. Jo Shapiro, MD, Explores Peer Support Implementation During a Crisis. Available at: https://www.ama-assn.org/practice-management/sustainability/jo-shapiro-md-explores-peer-support-implementation-during-crisis (accessed June 13, 2022).

APA Dictionary of Psychology. 2022. Stigma. Available at: https://dictionary.apa.org/stigma (accessed June 13, 2022).

Center for Creative Leadership. 2022. What is Psychological Safety at Work? Available at: https://www.ccl.org/articles/leading-effectively-articles/what-is-psychological-safety-at-work/ (accessed June 13, 2022).

Danna, K., and R. W. Griffin. 1999. Health and well-being in the workforce: A review and synthesis of the literature. Journal of Management 25(3). https://doi.org/10.1177/014920639902500305.

Doble, S. E., and J. C. Santha. 2008. Occupational well-being: Rethinking occupational therapy outcomes. Canadian Journal of Occupational Therapy 75(3):184–190. https://doi.org/10.1177/000841740807500310.

Edmondson, A. C. 2018. The Fearless Organization: Creating Psychological Safety in the Workplace for Learning, Innovation, and Growth. Hoboken, NJ: John Wiley & Sons.

Health Resources and Services Administration (HRSA). 2021. Health Workforce Strategic Plan 2021. Available at: https://bhw.hrsa.gov/sites/default/files/bureau-health-workforce/about-us/

hhs-health workforce-strategic-plan-2021.pdf (accessed June 13, 2022).

Litz, B. T., N. Stein, E. Delaney, L. Lebowitz, W. P. Nash, C. Silva, and S. Maguen. 2009. Moral injury and moral repair in war veterans: A preliminary model and intervention strategy. Clinical Psychology Review 29(8):695–706. https://doi.org/10.1016/j.cpr.2009.07.003.

Morley, G., J. Ives, C. Bradbury-Jones, and F. Irvine. 2017. What is 'moral distress'? A narrative synthesis of the literature. Nursing Ethics 26(3):646–662. https://doi.org/10.1177/0969733017724354.

National Academies of Sciences, Engineering, and Medicine (NASEM). 2017. Communities in Action: Pathways to Health Equity. Washington, DC: The National Academies Press. https://doi.org/10.17226/24624.

NASEM. 2019. Taking Action Against Clinician Burnout: A Systems Approach to Professional Well-Being. Washington, DC: The National Academies Press. https://doi.org/10.17226/25521.

National Institute for Occupational Safety and Health (NIOSH). 2016. Healthcare Workers: Work Stress & Mental Health. Available at: https://www.cdc.gov/niosh/topics/healthcare/workstress.html (accessed June 13, 2022).

National Institutes of Health (NIH). 2021. Cultural Respect. Available at: https://www.nih.gov/institutes-nih/nih-office-director/office-communications-public-liaison/clear-communication/cultural-respect (accessed August 31, 2022).

World Health Organization (WHO). 2007. Everybody's Business – Strengthening Health Systems to Improve Health Outcomes: WHO's Framework for Action. Available at: https://apps.who.int/iris/handle/10665/43918 (accessed June 13, 2022).

WHO. 2008. Closing the Gap in a Generation: Health Equity Through Action on the Social Determinants of Health - Final Report of the Commission on Social Determinants of Health. Available at: https://www.who.int/publications/i/item/WHO-IER-CSDH-08.1 (accessed August 31, 2022).

WHO. 2022. Mental Health: Strengthening our Response. Available at: https://www.who.int/news-room/fact-sheets/detail/mental-health-strengthening-our-response (accessed August 31, 2022).

INTRODUCTION

117th Congress. 2021. H.R. 1667 – Dr. Lorna Breen Health Care Provider Protection Act. Available at: https://www.congress.gov/bill/117th-congress/house-bill/1667 (accessed June 13, 2022).

Abbasi, J. 2022. Pushed to their limits, 1 in 5 physicians intends to leave practice. JAMA 327(15):1435-1437. https://doi.org/10.1001/jama.2022.5074.

American Academy of Orthopedic Surgeons (AAOS). n.d. COVID-19 Member Resource Center. Available at: https://www.aaos.org/about/covid-19-information-for-our-members/healthcare-policy-updates/ (accessed June 13, 2022).

American Hospital Association (AHA). 2021. Strengthening the Health Care Workforce. Available at: https://www.aha.org/system/files/media/file/2021/11/strengthening-the-health-care-workforce-II.pdf (accessed June 13, 2022).

Archambault, J. 2022. 10 State Health Policy Changes that should Outlive COVID-19. Available at: https://spn.org/blog/10-state-health-policy-changes-that-should-outlive-covid-19/ (accessed June 13, 2022).

Berg, S. 2021. Half of Health Workers Report Burnout Amid COVID-19. American Medical Association. Available at: https://www.ama-assn.org/practice-management/physician-health/half-health-workers-report-burnout-amid-covid-19 (accessed June 13, 2022).

Center for American Progress (CAP). 2020. On the Frontlines at Work and at Home: The Disproportionate Economic Effects of the Coronavirus Pandemic on Women of Color. Available at: https://www.americanprogress.org/article/frontlines-work-home/ (accessed June 17, 2022).

de Beaumont. 2021. 2021 Findings. Available at: https://debeaumont.org/phwins/2021-findings/ (accessed June 13, 2022).

Frogner, B. K., and J. S. Dill. 2022. Tracking turnover among health care workers during the COVID-19 pandemic: A cross-sectional study. JAMA Health Forum 3(4):e220371. https://doi.org/10.1001/jamahealthforum.2022.0371.

Hardy, L. J., A. Mana, L. Mundell, M. Neuman, S. Benheim, and E. Otenyo. 2021. Who is to blame for COVID-19? Examining politicized fear and health behavior through a mixed methods study in the United States. PLoS One. https://doi.org/10.1371/journal.pone.0256136.

Jones, G. M., N. A. Roe, L. Louden, and C. R. Tubbs. 2017. Factors Associated with Burnout Among US Hospital Clinical Pharmacy Practitioners: Results of a Nationwide Pilot Survey. Hospital Pharmacy 52(11):742–751. https://doi.org/10.1177/0018578717732339.

Kahan, S. and J. J. Avritt. 2015. Leading the Way to Scalable Social Change. Available at: https://visionaryleadership.com/christina-economos-leading-the-way-to-scalable-social-change/ (accessed June 13, 2022).

Khan, A., S. Jain, and V. Arora. 2022. The Demise of the Social Contract in Medicine: Recent Health Policy Changes Benefit Patients but Ignore Demoralized Health Care Workers. Available at: https://www.medpagetoday.com/opinion/second-opinions/96536 (accessed June 13, 2022).

Knoll, C., A. Watkins, and M. Rothfeld. 2020. 'I couldn't do anything': The virus and an E.R. doctor's suicide. The New York Times, July 11. Available at: https://www.nytimes.com/2020/07/11/nyregion/lorna-breen-suicide-coronavirus.html (accessed June 5, 2022).

Lai, A. Y., and B. P. I. Fleuren. 2022. Clarifying the concepts of joy and meaning for work in health care. Journal of Hospital Management and Health Policy. Available at: https://jhmhp.amegroups.com/article/view/6816 (accessed June 13, 2022).

Larkin, H. 2021. Navigating attacks against health care workers in the COVID-19 era. JAMA 325(18): 1822-1824. https://doi.org/10.1001/jama.2021.2701.

Maslach, C. 2018. Job burnout in professional and economic contexts. In Diversity in Unity: Perspectives from Psychology and Behavioral Sciences, edited by A. A. Ariyanto, H. Muluk, P. Newcombe, F. P. Piercy, E. K. Poerwandari, and S. H. R. Suradijono. London, England: Routledge.

National Academies of Sciences, Engineering, and Medicine (NASEM). 2019. Taking Action Against Clinician Burnout: A Systems Approach to Professional Well-Being. Washington, DC: The National Academies Press. https://doi.org/10.17226/25521.

National Academy of Medicine (NAM). 2022a. Clinician Burnout Crisis in the Era of COVID-19: Insights from the Frontline of Care. Available at: https://nam.edu/initiatives/clinician-resilience-and-well-being/clinician-burnout-crisis-in-the-era-of-covid-19/ (accessed June 13, 2022).

NAM. 2022b. Clinician Retention in the Era of COVID: Uniting the Health Workforce to Optimize Well-Being. Presentations from Rachel Villanueva and Kim Templeton. Available at: https://nam.edu/event/clinician-retention-in-the-era-of-covid-uniting-the-health-workforce-to-optimize-well-being/ (accessed June 13, 2022).

Nundy, S., L. A. Cooper, and K. S. Mate. 2022. The Quintuple Aim for Health Care Improvement: A New Imperative to Advance Health Equity. JAMA 327(6): 521-522. https://doi.org/10.1001/jama.2021.25181.

Patel, S. K., M. J. Kelm, P. W. Bush, H.-J. Lee, and A. M. Ball. 2021. Prevalence and risk factors of burnout in community pharmacists. Journal of the American Pharmacists Association 61(2):145–150. https://doi.org/10.1016/j.japh.2020.09.022.

Stone, K. W., K. W. Kintziger, M. A. Jagger, and J. A. Horney. 2021. Public health workforce burnout in the COVID-19 response. U.S. International Journal of Environmental Research and Public Health 18(8). https://doi.org/10.3390/ijerph18084369.

Templeton, K., C. Bernstein, J. Sukhera, L. M. Nora, C. Newman, H. Burstin, C. Guille, L. Lynn, M. L. Schwarze, S. Sen, and N. Busis. 2019. Gender-based differences in burnout: Issues faced by women physicians. NAM Perspectives. Discussion Paper, National Academy of Medicine, Washington, DC. https://doi.org/10.31478/201905a.

Thomas-Hawkins, C., P. Zha, L. Finn, and S. Ando. 2022. Effects of Race, Workplace Racism, and COVID Worry on the Emotional Well-Being of Hospital-Based Nurses: A Dual Pandemic. Behavioral Medicine. https://doi.org/10.1080/08964289.2021.1977605.

United Nations Human Rights Office of the High Commissioner (UNHR). 2020. Racial Discrimination in the Context of the COVID-19 Crisis. Available at: https://www.ohchr.org/sites/default/files/Documents/Issues/Racism/COVID-19_and_Racial_Discrimination.pdf (accessed June 17, 2022).

Yi, S. 2020. I'm an Asian American doctor on the front lines of two wars: Coronavirus and racism. The Lily, April 21. Available at: https://www.thelily.com/im-an-asian-american-doctor-on-the-front-lines-of-two-wars-coronavirus-and-racism/ (accessed June 13, 2022).

CHAPTER 1: PRIORITY AREA: CREATE AND SUSTAIN POSITIVE WORK AND LEARNING ENVIRONMENTS AND CULTURE

Accreditation Council for Graduate Medical Education (ACGME). 2019. CLER Pathways to Excellence: Expectations for an Optimal Clinical Learning Environment to Achieve Safe and High-Quality Patient Care. Available at: https://www.acgme.org/globalassets/pdfs/cler/1079acgme-cler2019pte-brochdigital.pdf (accessed June 13, 2022).

Amaya, M., B. M. Melnyk, B. Buffington, and L. Battista. 2017. Workplace wellness champions: Lessons learned and implications for future programming. Available at: https://nam.edu/wp-content/uploads/2019/09/Worksite-Wellness-Champions-Article-Amaya-Melnyk-Battista-BHAC-Journal-June-2017.pdf (accessed June 13, 2022).

American Association of Critical-Care Nurses. n.d.a. Beacon awards. Available at: https://www.aacn.org/nursing-excellence/beacon-awards (accessed June 13, 2022).

American Association of Critical-Care Nurses. n.d.b. Standards for establishing and sustaining a healthy work environment. Available at: https://www.aacn.org/nursing-excellence/healthy-work-environments (accessed June 13, 2022).

American Hospital Association. 2018. Culture of Well-Being. Available at: https://www.aha.org/system/files/2018-10/plf-case-study-avera-health.pdf (accessed June 13, 2022).

American Hospital Association. 2019. Well-being playbook: A guide for hospital and health system leaders. Available at: https://www.aha.org/system/files/media/file/2019/05/plf-well-655 being-playbook.pdf (accessed June 13, 2022).

American Medical Association (AMA). 2020. Joy in medicine health system recognition program. Available at: https://www.ama-assn.org/system/files/2020-10/joy-award-brochure.pdf (accessed June 13, 2022).

American Nurses Credentialing Center. n.d.a. Pathway to excellence program. Available at: https://www.nursingworld.org/organizational-programs/pathway/ (accessed June 13, 2022).

American Nurses Credentialing Center. n.d.b. Magnet recognition program. Available at: https://www.nursingworld.org/organizational-programs/magnet/ (accessed June 13, 2022).

American Nurses Association (ANA). 2022. Survey Shows Substantial Racism in Nursing. Available at: https://www.nursingworld.org/practice-policy/workforce/clinical-practice-material/national-commission-to-address-racism-in-nursing/survey-shows-substantial-racism-in-nursing/ (accessed June 6, 2022).

American Nurses Foundation (ANF). n.d. A nurse's guide to preventing compassion fatigue, moral distress, and burnout. Available at: https://www.nursingworld.org/continuing-education/online-courses/a-nurses-guide-to-preventing-compassion-fatigue-moral-distress-and-burno-12b2af6c/ (accessed June 13, 2022).

American Pharmacists Association and the National Alliance of State Pharmacy Associations. n.d. The pharmacist's fundamental rights and responsibilities. Available at: https://www.pharmacist.com/pharmacistsresponsibilities (accessed June 13, 2022).

American Society of Health-System Pharmacists. n.d. ASHP certified center of excellence in medication-use safety and pharmacy practice. Available at: https://www.ashp.org/pharmacy-practice/certified-center-of-excellence?loginreturnUrl=SSOCheckOnly (accessed June 13, 2022).

Barrett, E., N. M. Salas, C. Dewey, J. Ripp, and S. T. Hingle. 2021. A call to action: align well-being and antiracism strategies. ACP Internist. Available at: https://acpinternist.org/archives/2021/03/a-call-to-action-align-well-being-and-antiracism-strategies.htm (accessed June 13, 2022).

Bhatnagar, S., J. Harris, T. Hartnett, G. W. Hoagland, J. Ruff, M. W. Serafini, and D. McDonough. 2022. The Impact of COVID-19 on the Rural Health Care Landscape. Bipartisan Policy Center. Available at: https://bipartisanpolicy.org/report/the-impact-of-covid-19-on-the-rural-health-care-landscape/ (accessed August 31, 2022).

Dyrbye, L. N., T. D. Shanafelt, C. A. Sinsky, P. F. Cipriano, J. Bhatt, A. Ommaya, C. P. West, and D. Meyers. 2017. Burnout among health care professionals: A call to explore and address this underrecognized threat to safe, high-quality care. NAM Perspectives. Discussion Paper, National Academy of Medicine, Washington, DC. https://doi.org/10.31478/201707b.

Hu, Y.-Y., R. J. Ellis, D. B. Hewitt, A. D. Yang, E. O. Cheung, J. T. Moskowitz, J. R. Potts, J. Buyske, D. B. Hoyt, T. J. Nasca, and K. Y. Bilimoria. 2019. Discrimination, Abuse, Harassment, and Burnout in Surgical Residency Training. New England Journal of Medicine 381(18):1741–1752. https://doi.org/10.1056/NEJMsa1903759.

Institute for Healthcare Improvement. n.d. "What matters to you?" Conversation guide for improving joy in work. Available at: https://www.ihi.org/resources/Pages/Tools/Joy-in-Work-What-Matters-to-You-Conversation-Guide.aspx (accessed June 13, 2022).

KaufmanHall. 2022. National Hospital Flash Report: August 2022. Available at: https://www.kaufmanhall.com/insights/research-report/national-hospital-flash-report-august-2022 (accessed September 25, 2022).

Leape, L. L., M. F. Shore, J. L. Dienstag, R. J. Mayer, S. Edgman-Levitan, G. S. Meyer, and G. B. Healy. 2012. Perspective: A Culture of Respect, Part 2: Creating a Culture of Respect. Academic Medicine 87(7):853–858. https://doi.org/10.1097/ACM.0b013e3182583536.

Nasca, T. J., K. B. Weiss, and J. P. Bagian. 2014. Improving Clinical Learning Environments for Tomorrow's Physicians. New England Journal of Medicine 370(11): 991-993. https://doi.org/10.1056/NEJMp1314628.

National Academies of Sciences, Engineering, and Medicine (NASEM). 2019. Taking Action Against Clinician Burnout: A Systems Approach to Professional Well-Being. Washington, DC: The National Academies Press. https://doi.org/10.17226/25521.

National Academy of Medicine (NAM). n.d. Valid and reliable survey instruments to measure burnout, well-being, and other work-related dimensions. Available at: https://nam.edu/valid-reliable-survey-instruments-measure-burnout-well-work-related-dimensions/ (accessed June 13, 2022).

NAM. 2022a. Clinician Burnout Crisis in the Era of COVID-19: Insights from the Frontline of Care. Available at: https://nam.edu/initiatives/clinician-resilience-and-well-being/clinician-burnout-crisis-in-the-era-of-covid-19/ (accessed June 13, 2022).

NAM. 2022b. Clinician Retention in the Era of COVID: Uniting the Health Workforce to Optimize Well-Being. Presentations from Rachel Villanueva and Kim Templeton. Available at: https://nam.edu/event/clinician-retention-in-the-era-of-covid-uniting-the-health-workforce-to-optimize-well-being/ (accessed June 13,2022).

National Commission to Address Racism in Nursing. 2021. Survey shows substantial racism in nursing. Available at: https://www.nursingworld.org/~48f9c5/globalassets/practiceandpolicy/workforce/commission-to-address-racism/infographic--national-nursing-survey_understanding-racism-in-nursing.pdf (accessed June 13, 2022).

National Institute for Occupational Safety and Health. n.d. NIOSH safe patient handling and mobility. Available at: https://www.cdc.gov/niosh/topics/safepatient/default.html (accessed June 13, 2022).

National Institute for Occupational Safety and Health. 2020. NIOSH total worker health program. Available at: https://www.cdc.gov/niosh/twh/default.html (accessed June 13, 2022).

Perlo J., B. Balik, S. Swensen, A. Kabcenell, J. Landsman, and D. Feeley. 2017. IHI framework for improving joy in work. IHI White Paper. Cambridge, Massachusetts: Institute for Healthcare Improvement. Available at: https://www.ihi.org/resources/Pages/IHIWhitePapers/Framework-Improving-Joy-in-Work.aspx.

Prasad, S. J., P. Nair, K. Gadhvi, I. Barai, H. S. Danish, and A. B. Philip. 2016. Cultural humility: treating the patient, not the illness. Medical Education Online 21:30908. https://doi.org/10.3402/meo.v21.30908.

Shanafelt, T., and C. Sinsky. 2020a. Chief wellness officer roadmap. American Medical Association. Available at: https://edhub.ama-assn.org/steps-forward/module/2767764 (accessed June 13, 2022).

Shanafelt, T., and C. Sinsky. 2020b. Establishing a chief wellness officer position. American Medical Association. Available at: https://edhub.ama-assn.org/steps-forward/module/2767739?resultClick=1&bypassSolrId=J_2767739 (accessed June 13, 2022).

Shanafelt, T., J. Goh, and C. Sinsky. 2017. The Business Case for Investing in Well-Being. JAMA Internal Medicine 177(12):1826-1832. https://doi.org/10.1001/jamainternmed.2017.4340.

Sokol-Hessner, L., P. H. Folcarelli, C. L. Annas, S. M. L. Brown, L. Fernandez, S. D. Roche, B. S. Lee, and K. E. Sands. 2018. A Road Map for Advancing the Practice of Respect in Health Care: The Results of an Interdisciplinary Modified Delphi Consensus Study. The Joint Commission Journal on Quality and Patient Safety 44:8.

Wright, A. 2021. Rural hospitals can't find the nurses they need to fight COVID. Pew Trusts, September 1. Available at: https://www.pewtrusts.org/en/research-and-analysis/blogs/stateline/2021/09/01/rural-hospitals-cant-find-the-nurses-they-need-to-fight-covid (accessed June 13, 2022).

CHAPTER 2: PRIORITY AREA: INVEST IN MEASUREMENT, ASSESSMENT, STRATEGIES, AND RESEARCH

American Association of Critical-Care Nurses. n.d. Healthy work environment assessment tool. Available at: https://www.aacn.org/nursing-excellence/healthy-work-environments/aacn-healthy-work-environment-assessment-tool (accessed June 13, 2022).

American Medical Association (AMA). 2018. Organizational cost of physician burnout. Available at: https://edhub.ama-assn.org/steps-forward/interactive/16830405 (accessed June 13, 2022).

AMA. 2020. Cultivating leadership: Measure and assess leader behaviors to improve professional well-being. Available at: https://edhub.ama-assn.org/steps-forward/module/2774089 (accessed June 13, 2022).

American Nurses Foundation. 2022. Pulse on the nation's nurses survey series: COVID-19 two year impact assessment survey. Available at: https://www.nursingworld.org/practice-policy/work-environment/health-safety/disaster-preparedness/coronavirus/

what-you-need-to-know/covid-19-impact-assessment-survey---the-second-year/ (accessed June 13, 2022).

Brady, K. J. S., P. Ni, L. Carlasare, T. D. Shanafelt, C. A. Sinsky, M. Linzer, M. Stillman, and M. T. Trockel. 2022. Establishing Crosswalks Between Common Measures of Burnout in US Physicians. Journal of General Internal Medicine 37(4):777–784. https://doi.org/10.1007/s11606-021-06661-4.

Dyrbye, L. N., D. Meyers, J. Ripp, N. Dalal, S. B. Bird, and S. Sen. 2018. A pragmatic approach for organizations to measure health care professional well-being. NAM Perspectives. Discussion Paper, National Academy of Medicine, Washington, DC. https://doi.org/10.31478/201810b.

Dyrbye, L. N., D. Satele, and T. Shanafelt. 2016. Ability of a 9-Item Well-Being Index to Identify Distress and Stratify Quality of Life in U.S. Workers. Journal of Occupational Environmental Medicine 58(8):810-817. https://doi.org/10.1097/JOM.0000000000000798.

Dzau, V., D. Kirch, V. Murthy, and T. Nasca. 2020. Preventing a parallel pandemic — A national strategy to protect clinicians' well-being. New England Journal of Medicine 383(6): 513-515. https://www.nejm.org/doi/full/10.1056/NEJMp2011027.

Mayer, T., A. Venkatesh, and D. M. Berwick. 2021. Criterion-Based Measurements of Patient Experience in Health Care: Eliminating Winners and Losers to Create a New Moral Ethos. JAMA 326(24):2471–2472. https://doi.org/10.1001/jama.2021.21771.

Melnyk, B., and M. Amaya. 2018. Wellness culture and environment support scale. Available at: https://nam.edu/wp-content/uploads/2022/01/Wellness-Culture-and-Environment-782 Scale.pdf (accessed June 13, 2022).

National Academy of Medicine. n.d. Valid and reliable survey instruments to measure burnout, well-being, and other work-related dimensions. Available at: https://nam.edu/valid-reliable-survey-instruments-measure-burnout-well-work-related-dimensions/ (accessed June 13, 2022).

National Academies of Sciences, Engineering, and Medicine (NASEM). 2019. Taking Action Against Clinician Burnout: A Systems Approach to Professional Well-Being. Washington, DC: The National Academies Press. https://doi.org/10.17226/25521.

National Institute for Occupational Safety and Health. n.d. NIOSH Worker well-being questionnaire (WELLBQ). Available at: https://www.cdc.gov/niosh/twh/wellbq/default.html (accessed June 13, 2022).

Sinsky, C. A., A. Rule, G. Cohen, B. G. Arndt, T. D. Shanafelt, C. D. Sharp, S. L. Baxter, M. Tai-Seale, S. Yan, Y. Chen, J. Adler-Milstein, and M. Hribar. 2020. Metrics for assessing physician activity using electronic health record log data. Journal of the American Medical Informatics Association 27(4):639–643. https://doi.org/10.1093/jamia/ocz223.

CHAPTER 3: PRIORITY AREA: SUPPORT MENTAL HEALTH AND REDUCE STIGMA

American Psychiatric Nurses Association. 2020. COVID Resources. Available at: https://www.apna.org/covid-resources/?pageid=6685 (accessed June 13, 2022).

Bellini, L. M., M. Baime, and J. A. Shea. 2002. Variation of mood and empathy during internship. JAMA 287(23):3143-3146. https://doi.org/10.1001/jama.287.23.3143.

Brooks, E. 2016. Preventing physician suicide: Identify and support at-risk physicians. American Medical Association. Available at: https://edhub.ama-assn.org/steps-forward/module/2702599 (accessed June 13, 2022).

Buselli, R., M. Corsi, A. Veltri, S. Baldanzi, M. Chiumiento, E. Del Lupo, R. Marino, G. Necciari, F. Caldi, R. Foddis, G. Guglielmi, and A. Cristaudo. 2021. Mental health of health care workers (HCWs): a review of organizational interventions put in place by local institutions to cope with new psychosocial challenges resulting from COVID-19. Psychiatry Research 299(113847). https://doi.org/10.1016/j.psychres.2021.113847.

Butler Center for Research. 2015. Health care professionals: addiction and treatment. Available at: https://www.hazeldenbettyford.org/research-studies/addiction-research/health-care-professionals-substance-abuse (accessed June 13, 2022).

Fahrenkopf, A. M., T. C. Sectish, L. K. Barger, P. J. Sharek, D. Lewin, V. W. Chiang, S. Edwards, B. L. Wiedermann, and C. P. Landrigan. 2008. Rates of medication errors among depressed and burnt out residents: prospective cohort study. BMJ 336(7642):488-491. https://doi.org/10.1136/bmj.39469.763218.BE.

Fang, Y., A. S. B. Bohnert, K. Pereira-Lima, J. Cleary, E. Frank, Z. Zhao, W. Dempsey, and S. Sen. 2022. Trends in Depressive Symptoms and Associated Factors During Residency, 2007 to 2019: A Repeated Annual Cohort Study. Annals of Internal Medicine 175(1):56-64. https://doi.org/10.7326/M21-1594.

Federation of State Medical Boards (FSMB). 2018. Physician Wellness and Burnout. Available at: https://www.fsmb.org/siteassets/advocacy/policies/policy-on-wellness-and-burnout.pdf (accessed June 13, 2022).

Godfrey, K., and S. Scott. 2020. At the heart of the pandemic: nursing peer support. Nurse Leader 19(2):188–193. https://doi.org/10.1016/j.mnl.2020.09.006.

Guille, C., E. Frank, Z. Zhao, D. A. Kalmbach, P. J. Nietert, D. A. Mata, and S. Sen. 2017. Work-Family Conflict and the Sex Difference in Depression Among Training Physicians. JAMA Internal Medicine 177(12):1766–1772. https://doi.org/10.1001/jamainternmed.2017.5138.

Halter, M. J., D. G. Rolin, M. Adamaszek, M. C. Ladenheim, and B. F. Hutchens. 2019. State Nursing Licensure Questions About Mental Illness and Compliance With the Americans With Disabilities Act. Journal of Psychosocial Nursing and Mental Health Services 57(8):17–22. https://doi.org/10.3928/02793695-20190405-02.

Institute for Healthcare Improvement. 2020a. Conversation and action guide to support staff well-being and joy in work during and after the COVID-19 pandemic. Available at: https://www.ihi.org/resources/Pages/Tools/Conversation-Guide-to-Support-Staff-Wellbeing-Joy-in-Work-COVID-19.aspx (accessed June 13, 2022).

Institute for Healthcare Improvement. 2020b. "Psychological PPE": Promote health care workforce mental health and well-being. Available at: https://www.ihi.org/resources/Pages/Tools/psychological-PPE-promote-health-care-workforce-mental-health-and-well-being.aspx (accessed June 13, 2022).

Mata, D. A., M. A. Ramos, N. Bansal, R. Khan, C. Guille, E. Di Angelantonio, and S. Sen. 2015. Prevalence of Depression and Depressive Symptoms Among Resident Physicians: A Systematic Review and Meta-analysis. JAMA 314(22):2373–2383. https://doi.org/10.1001/jama.2015.15845.

McKay, D. and G. J. G. Asmundson. 2020. COVID-19 stress and substance use: Current issues and future preparations. Journal of Anxiety Disorders 74:102274. https://doi.org/10.1016/j.janxdis.2020.102274.

Melnyk, B. M., S. A. Kelly, J. Stephens, K. Dhakal, C. McGovern, S. Tucker, J. Hoying, K. McRae, S. Ault, E. Spurlock, and S. B. Bird. 2020. Interventions to Improve Mental Health, Well-Being, Physical Health, and Lifestyle Behaviors in Physicians and Nurses: A Systematic Review. American Journal of Health Promotion 34(8). https://doi.org/10.1177/0890117120920451.

Mental Health Technology Transfer Center Network. n.d. Provider well-being for behavioral health professionals. Substance Abuse and Mental Health Services Administration. Available at: https://mhttcnetwork.org/centers/mhttc-network-coordinating-office/provider-well-being (accessed June 13, 2022).

Muñoz, R. F., W. R. Beardslee, and Y. Leykin. 2012. Major depression can be prevented. American Psychologist 67(4):285–295. https://doi.org/10.1037/a0027666.

Nash, M. P., R. J. Westphal, P. J. Watson, and B. T. Litz. 2010. Combat and Operational Stress First Aid: Caregiver Training Manual. Washington, DC: U.S. Navy, Bureau of Medicine and Surgery. Available at: https://www.academia.edu/20978265/Combat_Operational_Stress_First_Aid_Manual (accessed June 13, 2022).

National Academies of Sciences, Engineering, and Medicine (NASEM). 2019. Taking Action Against Clinician Burnout: A Systems Approach to Professional Well-Being. Washington, DC: The National Academies Press. https://doi.org/10.17226/25521.

National Academy of Medicine and All In. 2022. 2022 healthcare workforce rescue package. Available at: https://www.allinforhealthcare.org/pages/2022-healthcare-workforce-rescue-package (accessed June 13, 2022).

National Alliance on Mental Illness (NAMI). n.d. Health care professionals. Available at: https://www.nami.org/Your-Journey/Frontline-Professionals/Health-Care-Professionals. (accessed June 13, 2022).

Shapiro, J. 2020. Peer support programs for physicians. American Medical Association. Available at: https://edhub.ama-assn.org/steps-forward/module/2767766 (accessed June 13, 2022).

U.S. Burden of Disease Collaborators. 2013. The State of US Health, 1990-2010: Burden of Diseases, Injuries, and Risk Factors. JAMA 310(6):591-608. https://doi.org/10.1001/jama.2013.13805.

World Health Organization (WHO). 2018. Mental Health: Strengthening our Response. Available at: https://www.who.int/news-room/fact-sheets/detail/mental-health-strengthening-our-response (accessed June 13, 2022).

CHAPTER 4: PRIORITY AREA: ADDRESS COMPLIANCE, REGULATORY, AND POLICY BARRIERS FOR DAILY WORK

Agency for Healthcare Research and Quality. n.d. NASA task load index. Available at: https://digital.ahrq.gov/health-it-tools-and-resources/evaluation-resources/workflow-assessment-health-it-toolkit/all-workflow-tools/nasa-task-load-index (accessed June 13, 2022).

American Medical Association. 2022a. Debunking regulatory myths. Available at: https://www.ama-assn.org/practice-management/sustainability/debunking-regulatory-myths. (accessed June 13, 2022).

American Medical Association. 2022b. Saving time playbook. Available at: https://www.ama-assn.org/system/files/ama-steps-forward-saving-time-playbook.pdf (accessed June 13, 2022).

Ashton, M. 2019. Getting rid of stupid stuff: reduce the unnecessary daily burdens for clinicians. American Medical Association. Available at: https://edhub.ama-assn.org/steps-forward/module/2757858. (accessed June 13, 2022).

American Occupational Therapy Association. n.d. Occupational therapy licensure compact. Available at: https://www.aota.org/advocacy/issues/ot-licensure-compact. (accessed June 13, 2022).

Centers for Medicare and Medicaid Services (CMS). 2020. CMS Takes Action Nationwide to Aggressively Respond to Coronavirus National Emergency. Available at: https://www.cms.gov/newsroom/press-releases/cms-takes-action-nationwide-aggressively-respond-coronavirus-national-emergency (accessed September 14, 2022).

Definitive Healthcare and Vocera. 2019. Cognitive Overload in Healthcare: How to Ease the Pain. Available at: https://www.definitivehc.com/blog/healthcare-cognitive-overload (accessed June 17, 2022).

Erickson, S. M., B. Rockwern, M. Koltov, and R. M. McLean. 2017. Putting patients first by reducing administrative tasks in health care: A position paper of the American College of Physicians. Annals of Internal Medicine 166(9):659-661. https://www.acpjournals.org/doi/pdf/10.7326/M16-2697.

Padden, J. 2019. Documentation Burden and Cognitive Burden: How Much is Too Much Information? Computational Informatics Nursing. https://doi.org/10.1097/cin.0000000000000522 (accessed June 17, 2022).

Rossetti, S. C., S. T. Rosenbloom, D. R. Levy, K. Cato, D. Detmer, K. B. Johnson, J. Murphy, M. Hobensack, R. Lee, E. Lucas, A. Moy, C. Sachson, J. Schwartz, J. Williamson, and J. Withall. 2021. 25x5 Symposium to Reduce Documentation Burden on U.S. Clinicians by 75% by 2025 Summary Report. Available at: https://www.dbmi.columbia.edu/wp-content/uploads/2021/12/25x5-Summary-Report.pdf (accessed February 27, 2023).

Sinsky, C. 2014. Team documentation: Improve efficiency of EHR documentation. American Medical Association. Available at: https://edhub.ama-assn.org/steps-forward/module/2702598 (accessed June 13, 2022).

Sinsky, C. 2015. Lean health care: Eliminate waste and spend more time with patients. American Medical Association. Available at: https://edhub.ama-assn.org/steps-forward/module/2702597 (accessed June 13, 2022).

Sinsky, C., and M. Linzer. 2020. Practice and policy reset post-COVID-19: Reversion, transition, or transformation? Health Affairs 39(8) https://doi.org/10.1377/hlthaff.2020.00612.

Sinsky, C. A., L. Daugherty Biddison, A. Mallick, A. Legreid Dopp, J. Perlo, L, Lynn, and C. D. Smith. 2020. Organizational Evidence-Based and Promising Practices for Improving Clinician Well-Being. NAM Perspectives. Discussion Paper, National Academy of Medicine, Washington, DC. https://doi.org/10.31478/202011a.

Smith, C. D., C. Balatbat, S. Corbridge, A. L. Dopp, J. Fried, R. Harter, S. Landefeld, C. Martin, F. Opelka, L. Sandy, L. Sato, and C. Sinsky. 2018. Implementing optimal team-based care to reduce clinician burnout. NAM Perspectives. Discussion Paper, National Academy of Medicine, Washington, DC. https://doi.org/10.31478/201809c.

CHAPTER 5: PRIORITY AREA: ENGAGE EFFECTIVE TECHNOLOGY TOOLS

American Hospital Association. 2018a. HCA healthcare program to streamline documentation for nursing. Available at: https://www.aha.org/system/files/2018-10/plf-case-study-HCA-health.pdf (accessed June 13, 2022).

American Hospital Association. 2018b. Just in time: EHR training at Atlantic Medical Group. Available at: https://www.aha.org/system/files/media/file/2019/08/alliance-cs-atlantic-medical-group-FINAL.pdf (accessed June 13 2022).

Alotaibi, Y. K., and F. Federico. 2017. The impact of health information technology on patient safety. Saudi Medical Journal 38(12):1173–1180. https://doi.org/10.15537/smj.2017.12.20631.

Ehrmann, D. E., S. N. Gallant, S. Nagaraj, S. D. Goodfellow, D. Eytan, A. Goldenberg, and M. L. Mazwi. 2022. Evaluating and reducing cognitive load should be a priority for machine learning in healthcare. Nature Medicine 28(7), 1331–1333. https://doi.org/10.1038/s41591-022-01833-z.

Jin, J., J. Reimer, M. Brown, and C. Sinsky. 2022. Taming the Electronic Health Record Playbook. Available at: https://www.ama-assn.org/practice-management/ama-steps-forward/taming-ehr-playbook (accessed February 27, 2023).

National Academies of Sciences, Engineering, and Medicine (NASEM). 2019. Taking Action Against Clinician Burnout: A Systems Approach to Professional Well-Being. Washington, DC: The National Academies Press. https://doi.org/10.17226/25521.

O'Shea, D. 2020. How health care providers can use technology to help improve patient care and their practices. Modern Healthcare, December 18. Available at: https://www.modernhealthcare.com/technology/how-health-care-providers-can-use-technology-help-improve-patient-care-and-their (accessed June 13, 2022).

Office of the National Coordinator for Health Information Technology. 2022. Trusted exchange framework and comment agreement. Available at: https://www.healthit.gov/topic/interoperability/policy/trusted-exchange-framework-and-common-agreement-tefca (accessed June 13, 2022).

Privitera, M., and K. MacNamee. 2021. Integrating patient safety and clinician wellbeing. [PowerPoint slides]. American Association for Physician Leadership. Available at: https://www.physicianleaders.org/articles/integrating-patient-safety-and-clinician-wellbeing

Sinsky, C. 2014. Team documentation: Improve efficiency of EHR documentation. American Medical Association. Available at: https://edhub.ama-assn.org/steps-forward/module/2702598 (accessed June 13, 2022).

CHAPTER 6: PRIORITY AREA: INSTITUTIONALIZE WELL-BEING AS A LONG-TERM VALUE

American Hospital Association. 2019. Well-being playbook: A guide for hospital and health system leaders. Available at: https://www.aha.org/system/files/media/file/2019/05/plf-well-being-playbook.pdf (access June 13, 2022).

American Hospital Association. 2021. Well-being playbook 2.0: a COVID-19 resource for hospital and health system leaders. Available at: https://www.aha.org/system/files/media/file/2021/02/alliance-playbook-2021_final.pdf (accessed June 13, 2022).

American Hospital Association. 2022. COVID-19: Stress and coping resources. Available at: https://www.aha.org/behavioralhealth/covid-19-stress-and-coping-resources (accessed June 13, 2022).

American Public Health Association (APHA). n.d. Prevention and public health fund fact sheet. Available at: https://www.apha.org/-/media/files/pdf/factsheets/200129_pphf_factsheet.ashx (accessed June 13, 2022).

American Society of Health-System Pharmacists (ASHP). 2021. Wellness with COVID: Contagious strategies to promote pharmacy well-being. Available at: https://nam.edu/clinicianwellbeing/wp-content/uploads/2022/01/Wellness-with-COVID-Contagious-Strategies-to-Promote-Pharmacy-Well-being.pdf (accessed June 13, 2022).

American Organization for Nursing Leadership. n.d. Leading through crisis: A resource compendium for nurse leaders. Available at: https://www.aonl.org/resources/leading-through-crisis (accessed June 13, 2022).

Barrett, E., N. M. Salas, C. Dewey, J. Ripp, and S. T. Hingle. 2021. A call to action: align well-being and anti-racism strategies. ACP Internist. Available at: https://acpinternist.org/archives/2021/03/a-call-to-action-align-well-being-and-antiracism-strategies.htm (accessed June 13, 2022).

DeChant, P. 2021. Building bridges between practicing physicians and administrators: improve physician-administrator relationships and enhance engagement. American Medical Association. Available at: https://edhub.ama-assn.org/steps-forward/module/2780305 (accessed June 13, 2022).

Farberman, R. K, M. McKillop, D. A. Lieberman, D. Delgado, C. Thomas, J. Cunningham, and K. McIntyre. 2020. The Impact of Chronic Underfunding on America's Public Health System: Trends, Risks, and Recommendations. Available at: https://www.tfah.org/wp-content/uploads/2020/04/TFAH2020PublicHealth-Funding.pdf (accessed June 13, 2022).

Frankel, R., and G. Beyt. 2016. Appreciative inquiry principles: Ask "What went well" to foster positive organizational culture. American Medical Association. Available at: https://edhub.ama-assn.org/steps-forward/module/2702691 (accessed June 13, 2022).

Godfrey, K., and S. Scott. 2021. At the heart of the pandemic: nursing peer support. Nurse Leader 19(2): 188-193. https://doi.org/10.1016/j.mnl.2020.09.006.

Institute for Healthcare Improvement. n.d. Conversation and action guide to support staff well-being and joy in work during and after the COVID-19 pandemic. Available at: https://www.ihi.org/resources/Pages/Tools/Conversation-Guide-to-Support-Staff-

Wellbeing-Joy-in-Work-COVID-19.aspx (accessed June 13, 2022)

Institute for Healthcare Improvement. 2020. Psychological PPE: Promote health care workforce mental health and well-being. Available at: https://www.ihi.org/resources/Pages/Tools/psychological-PPE-promote-health-care-workforce-mental-health-and-well-being.aspx (accessed June 13, 2022).

Institute for Healthcare Improvement. 2021. A guide to promoting health care workforce well-being during and after the COVID-19 pandemic. Available at: https://www.ihi.org/resources/Pages/Publications/guide-to-promoting-health-care-workforce-well-being-during-and-after-the-COVID-19-pandemic.aspx (accessed June 13, 2022).

Schmidt, M., and R. Aly. 2020. A Call to Action: Improving Clinician Well-Being and Patient Care and Safety. Health Policy Institute of Ohio. Available at: https://www.healthpolicyohio.org/a-call-to-action/ (accessed June 13, 2022).

Shanafelt, T. D., and J. H Noseworthy. 2017. Executive leadership and physician well-being: Nine organizational strategies to promote engagement and reduce burnout. Mayo Clinic Proceedings 92(1): 129–146. https://doi.org/10.1016/j.mayocp.2016.10.004.

Shanafelt, T. D., E. Schein, L. B. Minor, M. Trockel, P. Schein, and D. Kirch. 2019. Healing the Professional Culture of Medicine. Mayo Clinic Proceedings 94(8): 1556–1566. https://doi.org/10.1016/j.mayocp.2019.03.026.

Sinsky, C., T. Shanafelt, and M. L. Murphy. 2017. Creating the organizational foundation for joy in medicine: Organizational changes lead to physician satisfaction. American Medical Association. Available at: https://edhub.ama-assn.org/steps-forward/module/2702510 (accessed June 13, 2022).

Swenson, S. and T. Shanafelt. 2020. Cultivating leadership: Measure and assess leader behaviors to improve professional well-being. American Medical Association. Available at: https://edhub.ama-assn.org/steps-forward/module/2774089 (accessed June 13, 2022).

Uniformed Services University: Center for the Study of Traumatic Stress. n.d. Grief leadership: leadership in the wake of tragedy.

Available at: https://www.cstsonline.org/assets/media/documents/CSTS_FS_Grief_Leadership_in_theWake_of_Tragedy.pdf (accessed June 13, 2022).

CHAPTER 7: PRIORITY AREA: RECRUIT AND RETAIN A DIVERSE AND INCLUSIVE HEALTH WORKFORCE

Association of American Medical Colleges. 2022. Matriculating Student Questionnaire. Available at: https://www.aamc.org/data-reports/students-residents/report/matriculating-student-questionnaire-msq (accessed June 13, 2022).

Barrett, E., S. T. Hingle, C. D. Smith, and D. V. Moyer. 2021a. Getting through COVID-19: Keeping clinicians in the workforce. Annals of Internal Medicine 174(11): 1614–1615. https://doi.org/10.7326/M21-3381.

Barrett, E., N. M. Salas, C. Dewey, J. Ripp, and S. T. Hingle. 2021b. A call to action: align well-being and anti-racism strategies. ACP Internist. Available at: https://acpinternist.org/archives/2021/03/a-call-to-action-align-well-being-and-antiracism-strategies.htm (accessed June 13, 2022).

Bhatnagar, S., J. Harris, T. Hartnett, G. W. Hoagland, J. Ruff, M. W. Serafini, and D. McDonough. 2022. The Impact of COVID-19 on the Rural Health Care Landscape. Bipartisan Policy Center. Available at: https://bipartisanpolicy.org/report/the-impact-of-covid-19-on-the-rural-health-care-landscape/ (accessed August 31, 2022).

Boyle, P. 2021. Medical school applicants and enrollments hit record highs; underrepresented minorities lead the surge. Association of American Medical Colleges News. Available at: https://www.aamc.org/news-insights/medical-school-applicants-and-enrollments-hit-record-highs-underrepresented-minorities-lead-surge (accessed June 13, 2022).

Costa, D. K., and C. R. Friese. 2022. Policy strategies for addressing current threats to the U.S. nursing workforce. New England Journal of Medicine 386(26):2454-2456. https://doi.org/10.1056/NEJMp2202662.

National Academies of Sciences, Engineering, and Medicine (NASEM). 2021. The Future of Nursing 2020-2030: Charting a

Path to Achieve Health Equity. Washington, DC: The National Academies Press. https://doi.org/10.17226/25982.

National Academy of Medicine (NAM). 2022. Clinician Retention in the Era of COVID: Uniting the Health Workforce to Optimize Well-Being. Presentations from Rachel Villanueva and Kim Templeton. Available at: https://nam.edu/event/clinician-retention-in-the-era-of-covid-uniting-the-health-workforce-to-optimize-well-being/ (accessed June 13, 2022).

Pollack, R. 2022. Solving workforce challenges is key to advancing health. Modern Healthcare. Available at: https://www.modernhealthcare.com/opinion-editorial/solving-workforce-challenges-key-advancing-health (accessed June 13, 2022).

Shanafelt, T. D. 2021. Physician well-being 2.0: Where are we and where are we going? Mayo Clinic Proceedings 96(10): 2682–2693. https://doi.org/10.1016/j.mayocp.2021.06.005.

Sinsky, C. A., L. Daugherty Biddison, A. Mallick, A. Legreid Dopp, J. Perlo, L, Lynn, and C. D. Smith. 2020. Organizational Evidence-Based and Promising Practices for Improving Clinician Well-Being. NAM Perspectives. Discussion Paper, National Academy of Medicine, Washington, DC. https://doi.org/10.31478/202011a.

Smith C. D., C. Balatbat, S. Corbridge, A. L. Dopp, J. Fried, R. Harter, S. Landefeld, C. Martin, F. Opelka, L. Sandy, L. Sato, and C. Sinsky. 2018. Implementing optimal team-based care to reduce clinician burnout. NAM Perspectives. Discussion Paper, National Academy of Medicine, Washington, DC. https://doi.org/10.31478/201809c.

Warnick, A. 2021. Interest in public health degrees jumps in wake of pandemic: Applications rise. The Nation's Health 51(6): 1-12. Available at: https://www.thenationshealth.org/content/51/6/1.2 (accessed February 5, 2023).

Yong, E. 2021. Why health care workers are quitting in droves. The Atlantic. Available at: https://www.theatlantic.com/health/archive/2021/11/the-mass-exodus-of-americas-health-care-workers/620713/ (accessed June 13, 2022).